INTERNAL MEDICINE

ALSO BY TERRENCE HOLT

In the Valley of Kings: Stories

INTERNAL MEDICINE

A Doctor's Stories

Terrence Holt

LIVERIGHT PUBLISHING CORPORATION

A DIVISION OF W. W. NORTON & COMPANY

NEW YORK LONDON

For information about special discounts for bulk purchases,
write to Permissions, Liveright Publishing Corporation, a division of
W. W. Norton & Company, Inc., 500 Fifth Avenue, New York, NY 10110

For information about special discounts for bulk purchases, please contact
W. W. Norton Special Sales at specialsales@wwnorton.com or 800-233-4830

Manufacturing by Courier Westford
Book design by Lovedog Studio
Production manager: Anna Oler

Library of Congress Cataloging-in-Publication Data

Holt, Terry.
Internal medicine : a doctor's stories / Terrence Holt.
pages cm
ISBN 978-0-87140-875-4 (hardcover)
1. Holt, Terry. 2. Medicine—Anecdotes. 3. Internal medicine—Anecdotes.
4. Physicians—United States—Biography. I. Title.
R705.H65 2014
616—dc23
2014020125

Liveright Publishing Corporation
500 Fifth Avenue, New York, N.Y. 10110
www.wwnorton.com

W. W. Norton & Company Ltd.
Castle House, 75/76 Wells Street, London W1T 3QT

2 3 4 5 6 7 8 9 0

ACKNOWLEDGMENTS

SOME OF THE STORIES in this volume have appeared previously, in slightly different form. "A Sign of Weakness" and "The Perfect Code" in *Granta*, "Giving Bad News" (as "Bad News") in the *Boston Review* and (in abbreviated form as "Giving Bad News") in a literary supplement to the *Telegraph of India*, and "Orphan" in the *Boston Review*.

To William E. Holt, MD

Obiit 16 Jan 1994

Curse, bless, me now with your fierce tears, I pray.

CONTENTS

AUTHOR'S INTRODUCTION

Did you ask me why a surgeon writes?
I think it is because I wish to be a doctor.

RICHARD SELZER, 1976

T HIS BOOK IS THE STORY OF A RESIDENCY IN internal medicine. I wrote it over a period of ten years, beginning just after my own residency ended. The chapters appear here in an order that follows the trajectory of residency, from the first night on call to another call night some forty months later, by which time the narrator, no longer a resident, is out on his own, practicing as a hospitalist in a small town in the Midwest. I wrote this book primarily in an attempt to make sense of the process of becoming a doctor.

I first realized how much I wanted to tell this story on a day in March of my intern year, sometime between three and four in the afternoon. I'm at a nursing station, where three medical teams—each with its resident, interns, attending physician, medical students—and two or three consult teams of similar size and composition, along with nurses, CNAs, physi-

cal therapists, occupational therapists, speech therapists, the
chaplains, transport workers, dieticians, social workers, case
managers, maintenance workers, and probably others I've forgotten are all busy with the different things they do. Everyone
is talking at once. At any given moment, two or three of them
are trying to talk to me.

I'm standing in the middle of this roar and babble. My
pager is going off more or less continuously. The phones are
ringing, the unit clerk is crying out names (one of which, if
I could only hear him, might be mine) to come and take a
call. There are visitors, family members, and patients leaning
over the counters, each with some question, need, or piece of
information. From time to time the hospital PA system adds
to the din.

I'm worried about one patient who might be hemorrhag-
ing, another who could be going septic, and still another who
simply isn't getting better for reasons no one understands. I'm
worried that there may be yet one more on my list that I should
be worrying about, but try as I might I can't recall which one
that would be. It's unlikely I've eaten since five that morning.
My feet probably hurt. I know I'm tired. Details blur.

Still, I remember very clearly one day when I looked out
over this scene and said to myself: *This is not narratable.*

This was probably not the most useful thing I could have
been thinking at that moment. It was, however, true. What I
glimpsed that day was that the hospital is too manifold, too
layered, too many damn things happening one on top of the
other ever to get it down in its entirety. If there was any way
of doing justice to it, it would have to be through some kind

of condensation: by transforming it into a parable that could somehow imply the whole. I wasn't sure that was possible, either.

I realized only later how much I wanted it to be possible. I needed to understand how those years in the hospital had transformed me. This collection is not called *Internal Medicine* for nothing.

FORWARD A COUPLE OF YEARS. It's July, the month when everything changes: new residents arrive, others advance to another year, still others graduate, as I did this particular July. My memory of the transition is hazy. I celebrated the first several weeks by falling asleep wherever I sat down.

That month I also started writing these stories. There was no premeditation in this, and certainly no intention of producing the book you're holding. That moment in which I had recognized the non-narratibility of the hospital had produced, in a kind of delayed reflex, these attempts to get down some different kind of account of what it had been like. Not a record that accurately captured every relevant detail: I knew it was not possible to capture the meaning of residency that way. What I found myself writing instead was those parables I had imagined before, using them to identify what remained mysterious, and often troubling, about the process of becoming a doctor.

I understand that anyone picking up this book is probably hoping to learn something about what goes on in residency. The hunger to get behind the scenes of institutions that keep their inner workings hidden is powerful; this is especially so around medicine. I also wrote this book to satisfy that hunger, to give a truthful account of residency and the hospital. There are barriers, however, to giving such an account, limits on what a doctor is allowed to reveal. Patients have a right to privacy, of course. But there is something more than privacy at stake. You might change a few details: a name here, a hair color there, add a few years or drop a few pounds, give that one a different diagnosis and the other an Irish accent, and that's enough to conceal your patient's identity from the world at large. But that's not enough to respect the patient. As long as there's an actual, unique individual beneath that disguise, you're making a spectacle of somebody's suffering, and that's a line no one should cross. It's bad for the patient. It's not good for the writer, either.

This poses a challenge to a writer trying to offer a factual account of residency. Medicine without patients isn't a very useful story. This is why the patients in this book aren't based on specific individuals, no matter how disguised. They aren't "facts." They are at most assemblages drawn from a variety of sources, compiled from multiple cases, transformed according to the logic not of journalism but of parable, seeking to capture the essence of something too complex to be understood any other way.

In writing these stories I have drawn on what I thought and felt and generally did as a resident, but in re-creating experience as parable I have watched the narrator of these pieces evolve into someone else. He dealt with patients different from the ones I cared for, and did so, necessarily, in ways I never did. The mistakes he makes were not mine. He sometimes thinks and feels things, or fails to, in ways he would not be proud of were they generally known. But I like to think he does a pretty good job in spite of it all. He struggles with issues I struggled with, and with which every doctor struggles. He struggles differently from the way I did, but in the end he learns things that it took me much longer to figure out. In portraying his inner conflicts I have tried to get at what the hospital teaches us. I have tried, more than anything else, to be faithful to the inner life of medicine.

As to the externalities, the bits and pieces of special knowledge that constitute much of the appeal of medical accounts: I have tried to be accurate here as well, combining multiple hospitals into one that never existed, but in which, I hope, you will recognize the next hospital you enter.

While pressing life into story, I have tried to keep other agendas from creeping in. I don't think I have reshaped events simply to generate drama. Nothing happens in these pages that doesn't happen every day in a variety of ways in hospitals everywhere. I have had to simplify what defied narrative form, and alter or suppress whatever might have compromised the respect patients deserve. But in making sense of residency within the constraints of narrative form and human decency, I have hewed as closely as possible to the lived reality of the hospital.

Chapel Hill
November 2013

A
SIGN
OF
WEAKNESS

M Y FIRST CALL NIGHT AS AN INTERN, I RAN into Dr. M, one of the senior attendings, whom I had known for several years. "How's it going?" he asked me. I told him I was on call. "First call?" He smiled. "I remember my first call. About ten o'clock that night, my resident said to me, 'I'm going to be just behind that door. Call me if you need me. But remember—it's a sign of weakness.'"

I don't recall my response: I don't think I even had time to consider the story until evening, when the frantic milling about that makes up an intern's day had started to wind down. That day, we filled up early—three opportunistic pneumonias from the HIV clinic; a prison inmate transferred from Raleigh with hemoptysis, presumably TB, and a fever-of-unknown-origin.

Keith, the resident, whose job it was to direct me in my labors, felt this was a good day—his work was essentially done by five, as together we wrote admission orders starting the workup of the mysterious fever. He said to me, "I'm heading off to read. Call me if you need anything."

"But it's a sign of weakness, right?" I said, remembering Dr. M's story.

Keith laughed. "Right." And sauntered off down the hall.

Later, I was on the eighth floor, getting sign-out from one of the interns on the pulmonary service. It was almost seven—this was early in the residency year, and nobody was getting out before dinner. This intern was post-call, red-eyed, and barely making sense. Her sign-out list was eleven patients long. I don't remember any of it except the one: Mrs. B was listed as a *DNR/DNI 47yo WF w/scleroderma → RD*. "RD" meant "respiratory distress." The little arrow meant this was one possible effect of her scleroderma. I had never seen scleroderma before, and what it was, exactly, I could recall only hazily.

"She's a whiner," the intern explained. "Don't get too excited about anything she says." She paused. "I mean, if she looks bad, get a gas or something, but basically she's a whiner."

Whiner, I wrote down in the margin of the list.

I sat at the workstation for some time after that, running through lab results on the computer—the scheduled seven P.M. draw was still going on, so there was nothing new on the screen, but it calmed me to go through the exercise.

A nurse stuck her head through the door. "Doctor?"

I was still unused to people calling me that.

"Do you know the lady in twenty-six?"

I fished the sign-out sheets out of my pocket. "What's her name?" There were too many sheets. The nurse gave me the name and my eye fell on it at the same time. Whiner.

"What's her problem?"

"She says she's feeling short of breath."

"Vitals?" I heard myself ask, marveling at my tone of voice as I did.

The nurse pulled a card out of her pocket and read off a series of numbers. When she was done I realized I hadn't heard any of them.

The nurse read them again. This time, I wrote them down. Then I spent a minute studying them. She was afebrile, I noted. That was good. Her heart rate was 96, a high number I had no idea how to interpret. Her blood pressure was 152 over 84, another highish set of numbers that told me nothing. Her respiratory rate was 26—also high, and vaguely disquieting. Her O$_2$ sat—the oxygen content of her blood—was 92 percent: low, and in the context of that high respiratory rate not a good sign. The nurse was still looking at me. "I hear she's a whiner," I said hopefully. The nurse shrugged. "She asked me to call you."

The patient was alone in a double room. The light in the room was golden, the late sun of the July evening slanting through the high window. The face that turned to me as I knelt at the bedside was curiously unwrinkled. Her skin had a stretched and polished look, her features strangely immobile, the entire effect disturbingly like a doll's face. Her chest rose and fell, but her nostrils did not flare. Her mouth was a tight puncture in the center of her face. Only her eyes were mobile, following me as I moved.

"What seems to be the problem?" My voice had taken on a strange quality: tight, almost strangled.

"Are you my doctor?"

"I'm the doctor on call," I explained.

"I can't breathe."

I looked at her for a minute.

"What do you mean?"

"I can't . . . catch my breath."

I thought, but nothing brilliant came to mind. "Are you feeling dizzy?" I asked.

"No. Just. Short of breath."

I watched, counting. They were quick, shallow breaths, about twenty-eight of them to the minute.

I bent over her and placed my stethoscope on her back. I heard air moving, in and out, and a faint, light rustling, like clothes brushing together in a darkened closet. "I'll be right back," I said, and left the room to find her nurse. A few minutes later the nurse reported back to me. "Eighty-nine percent."

"Is she on any oxygen?" I should know this, I thought. I'd just been looking at her.

The nurse shook her head.

"Put her on two liters and check again."

Ten minutes later the nurse was back. I was in the doctors' workroom, looking up "scleroderma" on the Web.

"Ninety-one percent."

"That's better," I said hopefully.

The nurse shook her head. "Not on two liters. Not how hard she's working."

"You think she's working hard?"

The nurse smiled thinly. "Do you want to check a gas, Doctor?"

I smiled back, genuinely relieved that someone was willing to tell me what to do. "That's a great idea," I said. "Can you do that?"

"No. But you can. I'll get the stuff."

An arterial blood gas is a basic bedside procedure—the kind of thing third-year medical students are encouraged to learn. It involves sticking a needle into an artery and drawing off three or four ccs of blood. The reason a doctor has to draw it is that arteries lie deeper than veins. Even the relatively superficial radial artery—at the wrist, the one you press when checking a pulse—lies a good half-inch deep in most people, and sticking a needle in it stings more than a bit. I was not at that time very skilled at procedures—the arterial blood gas was about the limit of my expertise—but to my relief I had no trouble getting it: bright red blood flashed into the syringe. The patient bore this without a grimace, although by now I wondered if the skin on her face was capable of expression at all. Her eyes regarded the needle in her wrist.

"How are you feeling?"

"A little. Better."

I pulled the needle out, held a pad of gauze to her wrist.

She subsided into the bed. "But still. Short of breath."

I watched her. Twenty-six, twenty-eight. Shallow, the muscles at her neck straining with each one.

"I'll be back in a bit," I said, rising with the syringe in my hand. "Call if you need anything." But it's a sign of weakness, I echoed to myself. I hurried on down the hall, the echo following.

While I waited for the lab to process the gas, I skimmed over fifteen pages about scleroderma, a mysterious, untreatable condition in which the skin and organs stiffen. The most feared complications are cardiac and pulmonary. Some victims develop fibrosis of the heart early in the course of the disease and quickly die, as the accumulation of gristle disrupts the heart's conduction system. In the lungs, collagen invades the membranes where the blood exchanges oxygen and carbon dioxide with air: the lungs stiffen, thicken, and fail.

It is possible to get an idea of how this would feel. Putting your head in a paper bag is a dim shadow of it; thick quilts piled high come closer. The difference, of course, is that you can't throw scleroderma off. The bag stays dark; the quilts simply thicken, over years.

The blood gas was not encouraging. The numbers on the screen told me several things. Her blood was acidic. CO_2 trapped in her lungs was mixing with water in her blood to make carbonic acid. The acid was chewing up her stores of bicarbonate, which meant that her lungs were getting worse faster than her kidneys could compensate. The really bad news was the amount of oxygen dissolved in her blood, which at a partial pressure of fifty-four millimeters was unusually low, especially for someone getting supplementary O_2. Taken together, these numbers spoke of lungs that were rapidly losing access to the outside air.

I remembered a patient I had taken care of during an ER rotation a year earlier, an old lady with pneumonia. I had gotten a gas on her, too, and it had come back essentially normal. The attending had asked me to interpret it. "It's normal," I said. "And?" the attending replied, directing my attention to the patient gasping on the gurney. I looked at her for a moment. She was breathing about forty times a minute. "You're about to tube her," I said. "Right," the attending said, and did just that. A normal gas on somebody working hard is a bad sign. A below-normal gas on somebody working hard to breathe on supplementary O_2 is a very bad sign, especially if her chart carries the notation *DNI*. The letters stand for "Do not intubate." It's the patient's order to her doctors and it draws an inviolable line. No breathing tubes, no ventilators, no call to the ICU for help.

I hurried back down the hall to the room. The sun had set, leaving the sky a dim purple. The room was dimmer still, the patient's face a sheen on the white pillow, her chest visibly stroking from the door. I stood in the doorway for a minute, watching her, trying not to match her breathing with my own. Her face was turned to me. The eyes glittered.

"How are you feeling?"

"Not. So. Hot."

"I know," I said. "I'm going to get you some more oxygen." I reached for the regulator in the wall and cranked it up to six liters, the maximum you can deliver by nasal cannula.

The nurse appeared at the door. "Do you want me to call Respiratory?"

"Yeah," I said. "That's good. Call Respiratory." Respiratory therapists know all sorts of tricks: complicated masks that somehow squeeze more oxygen into room-pressure air.

I went back to the workroom and paged Keith. It occurred to me that I was displaying weakness. I told myself I didn't care.

He called back in a minute, cheery, calm. "What's up?"

I told him.

"She's DNR? You checked the chart?"

I set the phone down and found her chart. There in the "Consents" section was the legal form, witnessed and signed.

"Yeah. DNR/DNI."

"Well, that's it," he said. "If it's her time, it's her time. Just crank up her Os and give her some morphine. That's all you can do."

There was silence for a minute.

"Do you need me to come up there?"

"No. I'm on it. It's okay. I'll call you if I need anything."

"Okay. Have a good night."

It was eight-thirty. I went back to the patient's room. A respiratory therapist had arrived, bearing a tangled mass of tubes and bags.

"What do you want her on?" The tech eyed the woman in the bed speculatively. "Fifty percent?"

"Let's try that." I watched a minute as the tech unstrung his tubes, fitting valves together. The face on the pillow was blanker than ever now: she had closed her eyes. Without that glittering motion, her face looked as if it were simply waiting.

HALF AN HOUR LATER, the nurse found me again.

"Do you want me to do anything for twenty-six?"

"Like what?"

"She won't keep her mask on."

"Why not?"

"She says she's claustrophobic."

I threw my pen down on the desk.

THE EYES WERE OPEN again, looking out through the plastic skin. She was holding the face mask in her left hand, about a foot away from her face, as if restraining something that had tried to attack her. Her chest was still rising and falling too fast.

I went to the bedside and crouched beside her. The eyes slanted down with me, the head immobile on the bed. "I won't," she said, and pushed the mask into my hands.

"Why not?"

She shook her head. "Can't."

"Is it uncomfortable?"

"Suffocating. Can't."

I bit back an argument. "How about I give you something to help you relax?"

"Why?"

"You need the mask. You're not getting enough oxygen without it. If we can relax you a little, maybe you'll feel better about wearing it."

The eyes closed for a moment. "All right," she said.

I told the nurse to give her a milligram of Ativan and two of morphine, and to try to get the mask back on her.

Just after nine the nurse reappeared in the doorway of the workroom and shook her head.

"She won't keep the mask on."

I pulled myself to my feet.

The patient was propped up in bed now, leaning forward, her hands braced on her thighs to support her. The posture is called "tripoding"; it's something people do instinctively when they're having trouble getting air. Her shoulders were lifting and falling rhythmically with each breath. She was using what are called the accessory muscles, anything to help expand the ribcage with inhalation. It can buy you a little extra air exchange, but the price, in terms of exertion, is more than most of us can pay for very long. The mask lay in her right hand, hissing.

She didn't seem to notice me as I moved across the room; her gaze was straight ahead, intent on something. Each breath, I thought. Or perhaps something visible only to her through the far wall of the room.

"Mrs. B?"

Her gaze flickered my way, a brief acknowledgment, then back to her inner vigil, intent.

My first impulse was to ask her how she was doing. I stifled it. I reached out instead and took the mask from her. Her hand was stiff; the fingers yielded slowly. Her eyes turned toward me.

"Does this bother you so much?" I held the mask out.

She nodded and drew away. As if it could bite her, I thought.

"More than the way you're feeling now?"

Her gaze clouded a moment. Unfair, I thought. Arguing with a dying woman.

She nodded again.

I sat at her bedside, holding the hissing plastic coil, looking into the mask. Reluctantly, unwilling to place my mouth where hers had been, I fitted the mask to my face, pressed the vinyl against my cheeks. I took a breath.

There was only a smell of plastic, then a high, eerily open sensation of emptiness. I took a breath, feeling my lungs expand; a vivid impression of spaces opening everywhere. I found her looking back at me, the eyes from the depths of her immobile face dark and liquid and alive.

I took the mask off. "It makes you feel confined?"

She nodded, shrugged.

"Have you tried taking deep breaths?" I was still buzzing with the force of the oxygen; my lethargy and sleepiness were all gone. I felt ready to take this woman on and bring her with me to morning.

She looked at me only a moment before turning to the far wall again, shaking her head. It occurred to me that she probably couldn't take deep breaths.

I was still holding the mask.

"Did the sedatives help any?"

No.

"Would you like to try some more?"

Shrug.

I went to find the nurse. We doubled the dose of the Ativan. I watched, this time, as the drugs ran in, saw the relaxation I hadn't believed the stiff skin could show, the subtle slumping of the shoulders. I waited, and when sleep seemed about to take her I slipped the mask over her face. A hand stirred, rose a few inches, wavered, then fell to her lap; she settled back against the bed. I stood there beside her, holding the mask in place, watching. After a minute or two, we checked the pulse-ox: 94 percent. Her respiratory rate was settling into the mid-twenties. Hours of accumulated tension dissipated from my own chest. The nurse and I walked quietly out the door. "Keep an eye on her," I said.

I don't remember what time the next call came. Probably around two. I was back in the workroom, running blearily over the results of the one o'clock draw, fielding pages from the floor. There had been a shift change at midnight, followed by a flurry of pages from the new shift coming on with questions. There was a patient down on 3 West who was refusing his prep for a scheduled colonoscopy.

I heard a knock and an unfamiliar face appeared in the doorway. "Are you the doctor on call?" Shift change. I grunted something affirmative. "Do you know the patient in twenty-six?"

An uncomfortable sensation stirred in my chest.

"I got report on her," the new nurse said. "Do you still want frequent vital signs?"

"How's she doing?"

"I don't know. Do you want me to check?"

"Please," I said, and settled my head on my folded arms.

A HAND SHAKING MY SHOULDER. "Doctor?"

I stirred unpleasantly. My face was stiff. My sleeve was wet.

"I'm sorry to bother you, but that lady in twenty-six, she's not looking so good."

I sat upright.

"Her O$_2$ sat?" the nurse went on. "It's only eighty-two. And her rate is over thirty."

"Is she wearing her mask?"

"No."

"Christ." I was out of the room, stalking down the hall.

She lay in the bed, looking expectantly toward the door, the mask gripped in her hand. Her other hand went up as I approached, waving me away.

"Mrs. B," I called to her, pitching my voice as if into the distance.

The head bobbled for a moment, turned my way. The eyebrows were lifted slightly, but the skin above them was unfurrowed. The mouth was a hole air moved through.

"Mrs. B," I said again, willing her to look at me.

She did.

"You have to keep your mask on." It did not sound so idiotic when I said it as it does now.

She shook her head.

"If you don't do it," I said, reaching out to take the mask from her hand, "you're going to die." She made an ineffectual motion as I placed the mask over her face, looping the cord behind her head. Her hair was greasy with sweat. She reached up and placed a hand on the mask. My hand and her hand held it there. Did her breathing start to slow? I held the mask through one long minute, another. The nurse was a silhouette at the doorway. Another minute more, and I was sure the rate had fallen, the laboring of her shoulders lessened. To the nurse: "Let's check a sat."

Ninety-two percent. To Mrs. B: "There. That feels better, doesn't it?" She nodded, faintly, and seemed to settle into the bed. I let my hand fall away from the mask, crooning, "There, there." After five minutes pressing the mask to her face, my outstretched arm felt like wood. I reached behind her head to snug the cord.

She pulled the mask away. "I can't breathe. I don't want it," she gasped. "It's too tight."

And pulled harder until she snapped the cord in two.

I grabbed the mask and held it on her face. She reached up and clutched my wrist, and for a moment I thought we were about to struggle over it, but then she stopped and her hand fell away. Her eyes were fixed on mine.

The nurse was still at the doorway.

"Ativan," I said. "Two milligrams IV. And two of morphine."

Mrs. B still stared at me, her face remote and motiveless behind the mask. My arm was aching. Was I pressing the mask too hard? I eased up, fumbled with the broken cord, but the ends were too short to make a new one. Mrs. B didn't take her eyes off mine as the nurse reached for the port in the IV tubing. Just as the nurse's fingers caught it she snatched her arm away.

"No." The voice was a whisper.

The nurse turned to me, her expression stricken. "I can't, Doctor."

"What do you mean?"

"I can't force a patient. It would mean my license."

"She's going to die if she doesn't keep that mask on."

"Then get Psychiatry to declare her. But until then it's her decision. We can't make it for her."

Psych wasn't going to declare her. I knew that. It was her decision. I knew that. But I couldn't let it end this way. Surely I could make her see.

"Mrs. B," I said finally, "is there any way we can make this easier for you?"

"How about a bucket?" said the nurse.

My expression must have requested explanation.

"A face tent, they call them. It's open at the top. It works for claustrophobia. Do you want me to call Respiratory?"

"Please."

THE RESPIRATORY TECH ARRIVED after an interminable period during which Mrs. B refused again and again to wear the mask. Eventually we found a compromise. She would hold it a few inches below her chin. It bumped the pulse-ox to 88 percent. But her respiratory rate continued to climb. I couldn't tell if it was hypoxia or anxiety. A blood gas would have told me, but I was reluctant to try. I didn't know what I would do with the information. When the tech arrived and fitted her with the bucket, I stood at the door watching. It seemed to be doing something.

The next page from twenty-six came around four. I had gone into the call room fifteen minutes before, but the moment I lay down it was clear there was no chance of sleep. I lay rigid in the lower bunk, unwilling even to turn out the light, bracing against the sensation of my pager at my hip. My thoughts were an incoherent jumble: scraps of medical education—the innervation of the hand, the watershed areas of the mesenteric circulation, drugs to avoid in supraventricular tachycardia—none of which was relevant to any of the calls I had gotten that night. I was thinking of anything but the patient in twenty-six, two floors overhead. The next page was, of course, about her.

The nurse picked up on the first ring. "Doctor? I think you'd better get up here."

I was out of the door without a word.

The scene in twenty-six was superficially unaltered. But from the bed I was hearing small whimpering noises, rhythmic, paced almost to the beating of my heart.

She was sitting bent over, the exaggerated movements of her chest and shoulders making her head rise and fall, rise and fall. I counted, but lost track in the twenties, somewhere around half a minute. At least forty.

"Mrs. B?" I laid a hand on her shoulder. She didn't turn. Just the rapid rise and fall of the head. Her shoulder was clammy, her gown damp. Was she febrile? Was there something I'd missed? Should I have gotten cultures? Hung antibiotics? Was she having a PE? The body on the bed wasn't telling. Only the same carrier wave of distress, up and down, up and down. I looked to the door, where the nurse was standing. "Get Respiratory up here." She started to go. "And get me two of morphine."

The patient didn't resist this time. I don't know if she was even aware, but as the plunger went down on the syringe I could see a change in her; she settled and her breathing slowed. The pulse-ox, which had been in the mid-seventies, climbed up a notch or two, settled in the low eighties. I had no idea if that was something she could live with. I stood at the bedside and watched. Her respiratory rate was in the low thirties. An eye opened, swiveled around the room until it met mine. The mouth moved, no sound came out.

"Mrs. B," I said, and my tone was frankly pleading now, "you've got to let me help you."

The eye held my gaze for a long moment, the dim gleam of the nightlight streaking across the cornea. A hand made a brief sweeping gesture, fell. Away.

Somewhere in the course of the night I had developed a fixed idea: if I could get her to morning, it would be okay. I had no idea where that notion came from. Years later, after what seems like countless midnight vigils, the trust and hope of it chill me. But then I clung like a child to the thought of morning. In the morning, her primary team would be on hand; someone would know what to do. By the light of the morning, ill spirits flee. In the morning, it would be off my hands.

The respiratory tech was at the door.

"It isn't working," I said.

The tech didn't actually shrug. "You don't think you can tube her?"

"I can't," I gritted out. "DNI."

"BiPAP?"

"I can't get her to wear an ordinary face mask."

"Why don't you just snow her?"

It was a thought. She hadn't refused the morphine. I could try adding on sedation until she would let me put a mask on her—perhaps even a tight-fitting BiPAP mask, the next-best thing to intubation. It could be done.

"Yeah," I said. "Nurse? Bring me four of Ativan. And another four of morphine."

I knew the risk: knock her out too far and her respiratory drive would suffer; she'd lose her airway; she'd suffocate.

But she was going to die this way, too. I watched, holding my breath as the drugs went in, trying to remember the doses of naloxone and flumazenil that would reverse these, if I had to. *narcan   GABAA receptor*

Her breathing settled still more. Her eyelids fluttered and fell. "Get a mask on her," I said.

In a minute the tech had her fitted with an elaborate device that gripped her face like a diver's mask. There was no protest. The pulse-ox rose steadily to ninety, ninety-one, settled at ninety-two. I let out a sigh.

This time I did sleep. I must have, because my pager woke me from a dream of too many inscrutable objects, none of them fitting together, a puzzle I had to solve.

"Doctor? Twenty-six. She's fighting the mask."

SHE WAS SITTING UP, crouched as if clutching some secret to her chest. The mask was pushed up onto her forehead. Her shoulders rose and fell, rose and fell. She didn't look up as I entered; her gaze lay burning on the opposite wall.

The pulse-ox was eighty-two.

I laid a hand on her shoulder, could feel her bones working as it rose and fell.

"Mrs. B."

She shook her head.

"We've got to do something."

She shook it again.

"What can I do for you?"

Her hand waved me away.

I stood beside her, watching her breathe, for a very long time. She lay on the bed within reach of my outstretched hand, within the sound of my voice, but behind the wall of her fatigue and her breathlessness, sunk deep in her adamant gaze, she was unreachable. Unreachable by me. I wondered if she even knew I was still there, and felt suddenly a revulsion— not at her, but at my own presence in her room.

Her pulse-ox was eighty-two.

"Call me," I said to the nurse, "if she changes."

AROUND SIX A.M. I was sitting in the call room, trying to shake myself awake. My pager went off. It was the eighth floor.

The room was different now. Light was striking in through the window, a dozen rising suns reflected off the opposite tower. The room was bright and still.

Fast asleep, even comatose, a living body moves. The chest expands, the nostrils flare, the eyelids twitch; pulses stir the skin, and over all of these there hovers an inarticulate hum of life. But a dead body is only that: dead, a body, given over to gravity and decay. The muscle tone that lends expression to the face is gone; the face is slack; the skin gone gray-green with the absence of blood (underneath, if you turn it over, you will find pooled at the backside a livid bruise).

I went through the motions of declaring death. Her eyes

took my flashlight passively, the beam falling into the cloudy darkness of her pupils without a sign. I laid a stethoscope on her chest: only sporadic pings and creaks, sounds of a building settling in the night. Her flesh was cold, malleable, inert.

There were papers to fill out: organ donation, autopsy permission, the death certificate. I puzzled over "Cause of death," wondering just what process I had failed to reverse.

Respiratory failure, I finally wrote, *secondary to pulmonary fibrosis, secondary to systemic sclerosis.* The last line asked if any underlying medical conditions (diabetes, hypertension, for example) had contributed to the patient's demise. I looked at that a long time, and finally left it blank.

By the time I was done, the hospital had come to life around me. The intern who had signed out Mrs. B to me scratched the name off her patient list.

Keith, the resident, appeared on the floor just before rounds got under way. "How was your night?"

I told him. He listened to the story, pulled his lower lip, shook his head.

"You should have called me."

I flinched. "What would you have done?"

"Nothing," he said. "Just like you. There was nothing to do. But at least we could have done it together."

GIVING
BAD
NEWS

It's one of those icons of medical training, something you spend an afternoon discussing in the preclinical years and then gratefully forget, like community health or Medicare billing requirements. I don't remember anything we learned that day. All that stayed with me was a vague solemnity, a sense of having spent the afternoon in the middle of an Emily Dickinson poem—not one of the cheerful ones—and coming out of it about as wise for the experience. And so, as is inevitable with the lessons we tune out, it wasn't long before I learned this one the hard way.

He was a forty-three-year-old with pneumonia. I was an intern on the infectious-disease service. He belonged there only slightly more than I did. He did have pneumonia, but pneumonias aren't really all that infectious (most of them), and on a service crowded with HIV his presence was anomalous, more an accident of ER timing than a reasoned assignment from admissions. He had come up from the ER around two in the morning, admitted by the night float resident and

placed on my service. His story was unremarkable. He had
developed a cough, then fevers and shaking chills that bought
him a five-day course of azithromycin from his primary MD.
When he'd failed that, the primary had tried him on levoflox-
acin, a reasonably big gun. When he'd failed that, the primary
had sent him to the hospital "for further eval."

It's part of the nature of the hospital where I trained (as
it is with most teaching hospitals) that patients arrive without a great deal of documentation. In the typical community
hospital, if you're unlucky enough to find yourself hospitalized you at least have the consolation of knowing that your
own doctor, who presumably knows your medical history, is
going to be treating you. But admitting privileges at this facility are reserved for faculty of the medical school, who divide
their time between laboratories, clinics, and the floor. When
patients come here from what we generally call "outside docs,"
they usually arrive without any more medical information
than the patient can recall.

If the patient is well educated, articulate, and interested
in his health, that information can be complete—sometimes
too complete. But usually the patient is none of the above. I
wouldn't have had it any other way, but at times this complicated my attempts to understand what was going on. As with
this time. The history and physical on the chart didn't say
very much: the acute pneumonia, no other medical history
(not unusual in a forty-something man), a high school education, and a smoking habit. Not employed, living with family.
No meds.

As for the patient's current state of health, that was somewhat more complex. In addition to the pneumonia, which had him coughing up "bad phlegm" these past two weeks, he had reported some difficulty swallowing and a weight loss he could only quantify by saying that he'd taken in three notches on his belt since last Spring.

The resident said immediately, "That's not good."

I looked at him.

"Weight loss, difficulty swallowing, resistant pneumonia in a middle-aged male smoker," he said.

"Ah," I said, scanning the rest of the chart for a clue. The orders left by the night float resident included not the chest CT and bronchoscopy I had expected but an EGD—one of those gastrointestinal procedures where they stick a lighted tube down your throat and examine the inner lining of your stomach. "Ah," I said again.

The patient, an amiable, clueless fellow whose chief complaint when I met him after rounds was the absence of breakfast, looked better than his story sounded. Weight loss is a relative thing, after all, and until you get into the absolute end of the range, it usually doesn't show. He was a skinny man, who coughed once or twice with the weary, pained expression of a person who has coughed too much recently, and obligingly deposited the product in the plastic jar he'd been given for the purpose. The contents of the jar looked nasty, but then they always do. "When am I gonna eat?" he said, when he had finished screwing the lid back on the jar.

We explained about the EGD, and how he needed an empty stomach for the test. "Okay," he said. "And when's that gonna be?"

We told him that it was hard to say. It's always hard to say. This is more than usually distressing because most of the people waiting for the call are waiting with empty stomachs, and despite the low quality of the hospital food, breakfast is by far the best of it. Even dinner starts to smell pretty good when your roommate is being served and you're still waiting for your call to GI. So we're used to explaining to people why they can't eat: it's the kind of bad news that takes a while to sink in.

Mr. Jenkins spat disconsolately, as if he had a bad taste in his mouth, and we excused ourselves, promising to let him know as soon as we heard anything. Which of course we didn't, because we got busy with new admissions and no one ever tells the house staff anything anyway.

So when the number for GI procedures showed up on my pager it took me a moment to remember Mr. Jenkins. But that was all right because when I dialed it and heard the phone say, "GI procedures," they put me on hold before I could give my name.

Orville Shayne picked up. Orville, known universally as "Awful," was a first-year GI fellow from Chicago who had earned his nickname by being the most abrasive personality in the entire hospital. He was not averse to lessoning his betters now and then, and was entirely too eager to lecture the rest of us whenever possible.

"Who is this?" he demanded.

"It's Harper," I said. "You paged me."

"Harper. What are you going to do about your Mr. Jenkins?"

"What?" I replied, perhaps unwisely.

"Jenkins! Your Mr. Jenkins! The one you sent down here with"—he searched for a word sufficiently scathing—"*pneumonia.*"

"Look, Orville," I said, enunciating carefully, "is there a point to this? 'Cause I've got an admission down in the ER, and—"

"And you don't care about your Mr. Jenkins, is that it?"

This was starting to get me mad. "Do you want to tell me something, Orville?"

He snorted. "I suppose I'll have to, since I doubt you could interpret the pictures, which are in Mr. Jenkins's chart, by the way. Tell me," he said, "do you know what cancer is?"

What everyone wishes you'd get, I thought, but said nothing.

"As I suspected," Orville sneered. "Well, it's what your Mr. Jenkins has growing in his esophagus. Which is why he can't swallow, which is why he's losing weight, which is why he's got your *pneumonia.*" And then the line went dead.

Mr. Jenkins had esophageal cancer. It made sense. As Orville had so helpfully spelled out, it was the unifying explanation.

But what a nasty explanation it was. As it happened, I did know something about cancer, enough to know that esophageal cancer is an especially bad thing. It's not all that common; smoking and alcohol are probably risk factors. By the time it's diagnosed it is usually, as the oncologists say, out of the barn. Your odds of being alive five years after diagnosis are less than one in twenty. Starvation, hurried along by metastatic disease in the lung, liver, and brain, is the usual mode of death. You can try to put a rigid liner in the esophagus to hold it open.

You can try radiation. And, for the optimistic, you can try chemotherapy. It was a dismal future Mr. Jenkins had in store. And it was up to me, I realized as I turned from the phone, to tell him.

It wasn't, really. It wasn't, technically, up to me. The service I was on had a number of doctors with more knowledge and experience than I had. There was the resident, of course, still in-house. There was the attending, now gone home for the night, but he could certainly break the news in the morning—a lot better than I would, since he'd had the experience before.

I hadn't had the experience. And I needed it. And, to be strictly truthful, I wanted it. This was how we were supposed to learn. He was my patient, and I felt responsible for him. But, also, I wanted to be the one to tell him. It's something I can't explain—didn't understand then and perhaps would rather not understand about myself now. I hadn't had the experience, and I wanted to get it. So I squared my shoulders and marched down the hallway to Mr. Jenkins's room.

He was the only occupant of a double on the west side of the tower. Here on the sixth floor the view out the window was a sweep down the hill to the town, garish under sodium-vapor streetlights. The yellow glow from the street was the only light in the room. Mr. Jenkins was in bed, asleep. He was snoring unevenly, a little puddle gleaming darkly on the pillow beside his open mouth.

I stood at his bedside, listening to him breathe. Regular, unlabored, a little rattly, but basically the automatic tidal motion of a man in the middle of his life, the rhythm he had been maintaining from the moment of his birth. I stood there and listened to it, unconsciously holding my own breath for a long time until I realized what I was doing and drew a ragged breath out of the dark.

"Mr. Jenkins?" I said softly.

No answer.

"Mr. Jenkins?" I said again. This time I reached down and pressed his shoulder slightly. He stirred, and abruptly he was wide awake, astounded, raised on his elbow staring around the room.

"Wha'?" he said, or something to that effect. He was starting to pull back from me. In the darkened room, his eyes were enormous.

"Easy, Mr. Jenkins," I said in what I doubted was a reassuring tone. "You're in the hospital. Remember? I'm Dr. Harper. We met this morning."

Mr. Jenkins continued to stare at me as if I were a ghost, but he gradually subsided, muttering something I didn't catch beyond the tone of ebbing shock.

"Are you awake, Mr. Jenkins?"

He nodded, perhaps a more polite answer than the question deserved. And he lay there, still propped up on one elbow, waiting.

I realized that I had no idea how to proceed. I tried to think of something, but all I could come up with was the tune to "The Yellow Rose of Texas." It kept repeating itself unhelpfully, scattering my thoughts: beyond that, all of the advice from that long-ago dreary afternoon with Emily Dickinson had evaporated. And Jenkins was waiting. As if aware of my uneasiness, he was starting a shy, reassuring smile.

"Mr. Jenkins," I began.

He nodded at me encouragingly.

"I'm afraid I've got some bad news."

For a horrible ten or twelve seconds, the smile lingered on his face while the rest of his features abandoned it until it hung there in empty air.

"That test we did this afternoon?"

He nodded.

"It found a—a mass."

This wasn't right, I realized. I should just name it.

"They found cancer, Mr. Jenkins. That's why you've been having trouble swallowing. That's why you've been losing weight."

I stopped for a moment, unable to go on. In the silence that lay between us I recalled dimly that I was supposed to do this, supposed to give the patient time to grasp the news. Reassured by this, I let the silence grow.

Finally, his voice coming with effort, Mr. Jenkins said, "What's it gonna do?"

Patients have this terrifying ability to ask the question, the one of all others you don't want laid at your feet. I could feel myself start to choke. The easy answer, the immediate one, was *I don't know*, but I couldn't bring myself to say it—it would be too palpably a lie. Because I did know. We both knew. But I couldn't say that either.

I was wrestling with all of this, starting to hyperventilate, when I heard Mr. Jenkins sigh. "That's a bad question," he said. The ghost of a smile shimmered in the dim light. He settled back against his pillow, ran the back of a thin hand across his forehead. "Ain't nobody knows, do they."

"That's right," I said fervently. "But, Mr. Jenkins, I do know this. There are a lot of people in this hospital who can help you. The next thing that will happen is we'll present your case"— no, I thought, too legal—"we'll present you"—too formal— "we'll bring in a lot of specialists"—that was it: "specialists" had a reassuring ring—"and we'll help you fight this thing." Unless, of course, fighting wasn't what he wanted. What if he didn't want to fight it? I was just about to babble, I realized. "Would you like to see the chaplain, Mr. Jenkins?"

Mr. Jenkins lay back on his pillow with his left arm beside his head, fingers curled delicately as if waiting for something to fall into his palm. He closed his eyes.

"Maybe tomorrow," I said.

I don't know if Mr. Jenkins slept that night. I didn't, of course, being a green intern on call, prone to jump bolt upright at the sound of my pager, and feeling the need to go see every patient I heard about, whether the situation warranted it or not. But if I had been allowed to lie down for more than fifteen minutes at a stretch, I doubt I would have fallen asleep without Mr. Jenkins's expression hovering in the dark above me. I had nothing constructive to think about, nothing really to do about him. The machinery of oncology would be unleashed on Mr. Jenkins tomorrow, there would be a routine series of studies to go through, and his pneumonia would undoubtedly respond to the IV antibiotics he was getting every six hours. There was nothing in particular to think about at all. So it was only his smile that might have haunted me, if I had been available for haunting.

The next morning I was up and moving around, having gotten perhaps forty-five minutes of jumbled sleep and short-term memory disturbance somewhere between five and the sounding of my alarm at six in the morning. Rounds began at seven-thirty, and I had nine patients to see before then, giving me about ten minutes per patient, which even in my first week of internship was more than I needed to check the vitals, wake the patient, and do a quick exam. But I had set my alarm early with a thought to Mr. Jenkins, feeling that I would probably need more than ten minutes to see him this day.

I left him for last, of course, walking into his room with fully thirty minutes to go before rounds. The sun had risen by then, the world below his window blazing with color, each red leaf on the far hills distinct in the clear air. Mr. Jenkins was asleep, his pillow blotched with pink, green, and brown, his mouth slack, the same regular rising and falling of his chest.

"Mr. Jenkins," I said gently.

He roused more easily this morning, his eyes opening sleepily but without the terror of the night before. They opened, then opened wider, scanning the room quickly with an odd, stock-taking motion, as if he were in the habit of cataloging, every morning, the contents of his room.

He finished his survey with me, eyeing me with what I can only describe as a mild surmise. As he looked at me, uncertain, perhaps a little curious, I realized how deeply miserable I was to be standing before him. Not that I could think of any particular thing I'd done wrong. Just that it was miserable to be there, having to enter into it again.

"How are you?" I said gently.

"I'm not bad," he said. "Been coughing up a bit, not so bad."

"Good," I said. I moved to the bedside, sank down in the chair, and took a breath.

Mr. Jenkins regarded me, and his gaze as I looked back at him took another one of those curious sweeps around the room, returning to me. His expression was open, friendly, almost perky.

"So tell me," I began. "Have you been thinking?"

Jenkins looked puzzled. "Thinking," he said noncommittally.

I waited, but he had nothing more to add.

"Yes," I said. "About . . ."

He elevated his eyebrows helpfully. "About?"

"You know."

"Oh," he said. The eyebrows settled, pressed down by a pair of deep furrows. "I don't know," he added after a while.

"I understand," I said. "It's a lot to take in."

"Yeah," he said. And then: "A lot."

"Yeah," I agreed.

We sat there for a little while longer, thinking about a lot together.

"What do *you* think?" he said finally.

"Me?" I squeaked. I was suddenly aware of the time. "It's not really what I think," I began. "Is it?"

If I was thinking he was going to help me out, I was wrong. Mr. Jenkins stared back at me across his bedclothes, his hands lying on top of the cotton blanket as inert as old socks, the expression on his face an open blank. Open and blank. Not frightened. Not worried. Not remotely comprehending what had me so solemn and upset.

"Mr. Jenkins?" I said finally.

The eyebrows lifted a half degree.

"You do know what we're talking about, don't you?"

No change at all. For an instant I hoped wildly that this was cultural, this was some strange thing that came from class or poverty that I wasn't getting, and I shouldn't mess with it. But it was too late for that.

"We're talking about your diagnosis," I said slowly. "You remember, don't you?"

Now the eyes did begin to widen, the whites showing between the irises and the upper lids.

"What I told you last night? About the cancer?"

The face went stricken.

"I've got cancer?" It was a hoarse whisper, twisting upward at the end.

"It's in your throat," I said, pointing to mine. "It's why you're having so much trouble swallowing."

He blinked at that. "I got cancer," he mumbled, looking inward for a moment, nodding again. Then back at me. "What's it gonna do?"

I told the story on rounds. After the recitation of vital signs and exam findings, I added a brief anecdote describing his reaction to the news. The attending nodded and shook his head. "You'll get used to this," he told me. "We get so hardened to other people's bad news. It's hard to remember what a shock it is to them. Give him time to get used to it."

THEY SAY THAT TIME assuages, and time was, for once, something we had to give. This was Friday; we had an entire weekend before the breakneck rhythm of the hospital took hold of Mr. Jenkins and clutched him to itself. The pieces of aberrant flesh that were snipped from his mass in the GI-procedures suite spent the weekend absorbing stains in the pathology lab. On Monday, Tuesday at the latest, we would have the definitive diagnosis. In the interim there were some things we could get done despite the weekend, and we went ahead and did them—CT scans, chiefly, looking for possible metastases. The goal was to assess the spread of his disease—to "stage" him—and to assemble every other relevant bit of data in time for the multidisciplinary oncology conference that met in the cancer center every Wednesday. There, about two dozen representatives from medicine, surgery, pathology, radiology, pharmacology, and probably theology reviewed the dozen or so new cancer cases that had come up in the previous week, with the goal of arriving at a consensus and a plan.

But for now, Mr. Jenkins had time, a quiet weekend in a room with a view of Fall descending over the Piedmont.

Having been on call on a Thursday, I was facing my Golden Weekend—the once-a-month privilege accorded interns: two consecutive days off. I spent them with my family. Sixty hours together. On my return early Monday morning to the upper floors of the hospital I had a sensation of having been out of the action a very long time. Many of the patients I had been taking care of on Friday were gone, having been discharged by my resident over the weekend. Mr. Jenkins, naturally, was not one of those. I found him in his room, sleeping, a towel wrapped carefully around his head.

One of the things I passionately hate about my job is that it requires me to disturb people's sleep, sick people who have managed, against the odds, to achieve some measure of oblivion. As I've grown older in the profession, I have become less conscientious—I often let patients sleep—but in those days I was conscientious to a fault. I roused each patient so that he or she could bear witness to the events since I had seen them last.

It was no different with Mr. Jenkins. I called his name from the doorway, softly, then as I moved to the bedside called again, using the same tone I use when waking my children. I pressed briefly on his shoulder and called his name again. This time he stirred and peeled himself a peephole in the towel.

"Whazzat?"

"Hi, Mr. Jenkins," I said softly. "It's Dr. Harper." I paused to let that sink in. "How was your weekend?"

The eye goggled around the room in the same odd stock-taking I'd seen the first morning, before returning to settle on me.

"Okay," he said softly. Then the eye inspected again. It seemed to be looking for something.

"Did you get any visitors?"

"No." The eye was still, some small creature sulking in its hole.

"I'm sorry," I said, and I meant it, too, thinking about him spending the weekend with nothing to think about but his dismal prognosis. If there's any time you want family around, it's when you're looking at something like that.

I said as much to Mr. Jenkins. I can't remember the exact words I used. I don't suppose they mattered, because I found that eye of his staring at me and growing rounder until the towel came off his face and he was lying there looking at me with horror everywhere in the bed around him.

"You say *what*?"

Then it was my turn to stare back at him, and maybe there was a little horror in my face, too. All I know was that for a long time we stared at each other as if each found the other completely incomprehensible.

But it was up to me to break out of it first, and I did.

"Your . . . cancer," I said.

He tried to say something but it strangled to a whisper.

"Do you mean you don't remember?"

He shook his head.

"Well." I stopped short, at a loss for words. "There are some things the brain just doesn't want to hold on to," I said finally.

He was simply staring at me. Clearly I wasn't connecting.

"Would you like me to tell you again?"

After a long pause he nodded. I took a breath, and with a fugitive sense that this wasn't getting easier with repetition, I told him the story again. He seemed to take it in. He asked the same terrible questions. I had the same terrible lack of answers. And we left it at that.

I walked out of the room feeling shaken. It was partly the sheer rigor of it, having to tell again the story I'd never wanted to tell the first time. Or, okay, had wanted to tell, but only once. Was I being punished by some obscure hospital devil, forced for my sin of pride to experience again and again just what we do when we give bad news? I had a brief vision of myself as some kind of Kübler-Rossian version of the *Flying Dutchman*, doomed to wander the hospital forever in an unending struggle with denial. But that wasn't it, not really. Mr. Jenkins wasn't playing by the rules. Say what you want about denial, there was something else going on.

I tried to convey this on rounds, when we arrived at Mr. Jenkins's door. I made a hash of it, of course, trying to wedge in between the morning's lab results and the scheduled pulmonary function tests some ghostly aperçu I couldn't articulate even to myself.

The attention span of a team on rounds is short at the best of times. I could tell I'd lost the interest of the resident. The other intern, scheduled for clinic in the afternoon and desperate to be done rounding, looked at me with something that fell just short of hatred. The med students stood apart in some shared goofiness. Only the attending was still looking at me, his expression a tolerant mixture of amusement and minimal curiosity.

"What do you think it is?" he asked me.

"I don't know," I confessed, feeling miserable that I was making an ass of myself. But Mr. Jenkins wasn't playing by the rules.

What were the rules? I found myself wondering later. I had reached one of those random dead spells in the admitting day. I was at the workstation, going over sign-out sheets left by the three other interns whose patients I was covering

overnight. *Cx if spike*; *lasix 80 for SOB*; *Call VIR if HCT↓*:
I had several pages of helpful hints from my peers on how to
manage their patients' likely misadventures. But there was
no similar advice for how to deal with Mr. Jenkins. *Give him
the bad news* until he finally believes it, because he has to.
Make him do it until he gets it right. Isn't that right? Wasn't
I doing it right?

Naturally, the next morning I saved Mr. Jenkins's room for
last on my early rounds, and knocked on the door with dread.
I heard him hawk up something wet, spit, and then say, "Come
in." At the sound of his voice—a little guarded but otherwise
sprightly—my heart sank.

He was sitting up, looking around him as if puzzled by his
surroundings.

I stood in the doorway, a profound reluctance holding me.

"Hi," he said. I was suddenly aware that Mr. Jenkins was
shy.

"Hi," I said back. I am usually shy too. This morning more
so.

We held our positions for a long minute.

"Do I know you?" he asked.

The question hit me hard. The room took a sudden surge
toward me, settling in a series of uneasy swells as I tried to
absorb what he'd said. Not that I expect all my patients to
know my name, or even recognize me for the most part—all
those white coats. In most cases the acquaintance is all too
brief, too casual. But Mr. Jenkins and I had accumulated some
history.

I eased into the room, moving carefully as one might around

a nervous beast, keeping my eyes on his as they followed my progress toward the bed.

"Don't you?" I said as I crouched beside him.

He stared at me with a slowly dawning recognition that as I watched grew into horror.

"You know me, don't you?" I said quietly. What was this? Some kind of conversion disorder? A hysterical amnesia? "You've seen me before, haven't you?"

Jenkins's head wobbled uncertainly between yes and no.

"I'm Dr. Harper," I said quietly. "And you're here because—"

Jenkins suddenly whipped his bedsheet over his head, clutching it there like a Halloween ghost. The ghost shook its head emphatically and let out a low moan.

"Oh, God. It happened. It happened, didn't it."

"What happened?" I asked.

He threw off the sheet, and his gaze scattered around the room, taking in the surroundings one more time. "I knew it," he sobbed. "I knew it."

This was progress, I thought, triumphantly—and felt immediately guilty as I realized how stricken he looked, staring around at the walls as though he expected them to fall on him.

But I was making progress. Carefully, I prodded him. "Knew what?"

He moaned. "It's the crazy house. It's the crazy house, isn't it?" He buried his face in the sheet again.

Whatever I'd been planning to say up to that point vanished in an instant, leaving me flat-footed. "Did I"— the voice came muffled through the sheet—"*do* something?" The face appeared, eyes reconnoitering nervously above the sheet as the voice dropped confidentially. "It wasn't murder, was it? I didn't—"

"No," I said, a little louder than I'd intended. "You didn't—"

"Oh, thank God," he said. "Thank God. As long as I didn't—you don't know," he said soulfully.

"Don't know what?" There was a lot I didn't know, but Mr. Jenkins seemed to have something particular in mind. As for me, my head was swimming.

Jenkins had recovered some of his usual equanimity. The look he was giving me now was downright cagey.

"Don't you know?" he said.

I shook my head. "No, Mr. Jenkins. I don't know. What?"

"What it's like. Waking up every day."

I took a wild guess. "With cancer?"

He turned on me. "What?"

"With cancer," I said, perhaps a little more brusquely than I'd intended. "Waking up every day with cancer. Knowing about it, I mean. Waking up that way. Knowing. With cancer."

The expression he gave me had nothing to do with my stumbling delivery.

"*What?*"

"Cancer." Repressing panic, I might have been shouting. "You've got cancer."

A long silence, broken by the sound of his breathing. It was getting louder and louder.

"*What kind of doctor are you?*" He was half out of bed, shaking a double-handful of bedsheet in my face. I started to back away.

"What kind of doctor are you?" he demanded again. "Coming in here and telling me something like that? Is that how you tell somebody that kind of thing? You're lying! You don't tell me that! You don't come in here and tell me that kind of shit! Get out! Get out of here!"

By that time I was already out the door. I could hear his shouting all the way down the hall.

How I got through rounds that morning, I'll never know. Maybe the rest of the team attributed my zombie-like demeanor to the rigors of a rough call night, I don't know. All I remember was that I watched, as if from an indefinite distance, as the knot of us worked our way around the floor, measuring with growing dread the approach to Jenkins's room and the moment when I was going to have to face him again. I was listening, too, for the sound of shouts from that direction, wondering if there was any way I could avoid going in that room again. Perhaps I could simply make a run for it, before the moment when the patient reported that I had come in that morning and abused him. What kind of doctor was I?

Helpless in the grip of forces I did not understand, there I stood again finally, at the door of Jenkins's room, reciting by rote his vital signs that morning, exam findings, the results of yesterday's tests. I ground down. There was a pause.

"And?" the attending said mildly.

I might have jumped.

"Any progress?"

"Progress?"

Impatience. "You were going to work with him. On his diagnosis. I thought he was having trouble with it. Any luck?"

I shook my head dumbly.

The attending didn't wait, only nodded and swept open the door to Jenkins's room. I took a deep breath and followed.

Jenkins was back in bed, looking peaceful enough. The television set was on. Katie Couric was interviewing a woman who looked just like Katie Couric. Mr. Jenkins was rapt.

We all stood for a moment looking at Mr. Jenkins. As the interview cut to a commercial, Jenkins's gaze turned slowly to us, widening to take in the small crowd wedging into his room. I recognized his expression—the same cagey inventory, twice around his surroundings, the same poker face settling down.

"Hi," he said shyly.

"Good morning, Mr. Jenkins," the attending said.

We all stood and looked at each other some more.

"Mr. Jenkins?"

"Yeah?"

"Would you mind if we asked you some questions?"

"Uh-uh." The commercials were over. Mr. Jenkins's vision was starting to stray again.

"Can you tell us why you're here?"

A brief inner consultation. "Sure." He leaned over and spat into the wastecan. "This," he said. "It's been going on for a while."

"And?"

"Tastes nasty." He made a face.

"Anything else?"

"Well, yeah. I got this sore throat." He laid a hand on his chest. "It really doesn't feel good. I was wondering if maybe I got some kind of ulcer. You know? 'Cause my brother, he's got ulcers bad. I was wondering if maybe they run in the family? 'Cause if they do, maybe that's what I got."

"You've got a brother, Mr. Jenkins?"

It was news to me. It was news to all of us. As we left the room, the attending muttered to me, "Call psych. And call the brother."

Easier said than done, of course. When asked for his brother's phone number, Mr. Jenkins agreeably recited a string of digits that connected me with a fax machine. When asked again, he wanted to know why I wanted to talk to his brother. "It's about your ulcers," I said simply. I was tired. He gave me another string of numbers, which offered the mechanical advice that the number was not in service. On my third trip back I got as far as Jenkins's door before I realized that the two numbers he'd given me were in different area codes. I spun on my heel, went back to the nursing station, and pulled his chart.

"MR. JENKINS," I ASKED, "where do you live?"

"Lumberton."

His chart gave an address in Fayetteville.

"How long have you lived there?"

The expression went cagey again. The eyes narrowed. "Fifteen years. Yeah. Fifteen. Right out of high school."

I gave that some thought. This was a forty-three-year-old male with pneumonia. Somewhere along the way Mr. Jenkins had misplaced a decade.

"Mr. Jenkins," I asked slowly. "Can you tell me what year this is?"

"Sure."

We looked at each other for a minute.

"What year is it?"

"What year? Hmm. It's—I'm not too good with numbers. It's a leap year, isn't it?"

It was in fact a leap year.

"Can you tell me who the president is?"

"I don't follow politics. It's a dirty business. But sure." He looked cagey again. "It's Bush. George Bush."

I looked at him, feeling beaten. He looked back at me. A brief standoff, then he coughed self-consciously. The cough turned into a real one, and when he'd recovered his breath, he looked at me again. "What were we talking about?"

We did consult psych. They came by and gave the diagnosis of Wernicke-Korsakoff dementia. He'd completely fried his short-term memory with too much alcohol. By that time, I'd managed to track down the brother, who confirmed what I'd finally recognized, and a little bit more. It had been several years since Charles Jenkins had seen his brother, but he gave the essential outlines of the story. Mr. Jenkins had been in the Navy. He was in fact forty-three years old. But between the ages of eighteen and thirty-eight, he'd hadn't been sober more than three days at a time. The brother said this with a weary resignation in which I tried but failed to hear a trace of bitterness. I wanted to hear the rest of the story, but Charles Jenkins cut it short.

"When can he come home?"

———————

TWO DAYS LATER. Mr. Jenkins, his cancer thoroughly staged and determined beyond any hope of cure, sits peacefully in the recliner in his room. He is dressed in street clothes. Sunlight is streaming in over his shoulder, he's breathing comfortably, and the television set is tuned to one of the two hospital channels, which is showing a locally produced documentary about dialysis. When I go in to see him one last time, Mr. Jenkins is watching, rapt. I realize I'm almost looking forward to introducing myself again, if only to say goodbye. And for a moment I watch him, and find myself equally rapt at the sight of him: sick, dying, and eternally unaware. For a moment I am almost envious.

The feeling passes, replaced by a kind of nostalgia. He'll forget me again as soon as I'm gone. I'll never learn from his account of me what kind of doctor I am. But that's not it: I am tantalized by the sense that I've missed something here. I thought I was giving him bad news. The bad news wasn't his, but mine.

Out at the nursing station, I pick out of the general hubbub a nurse's voice speaking my name and the words "over there," and through the doorway see a man looking my way.

The family resemblance is strong. "I'm Charles Jenkins," the man says. He looks past me into the room. At my back I hear a sudden cry.

The reunion is a happy one. I leave them there, edging out of the room as I've edged out of so many, leaving the family to gather up the plastic bags of personal belongings, medications, paperwork with discharge instructions. My last memory of Thomas Jenkins is of him looking up from the chair, sunlight surrounding him, his face alight in the recognition of one of the few faces in the world he can still remember.

I like to think of him that way. That way, and no other. I only wish I could hold myself so finally aloof from time.

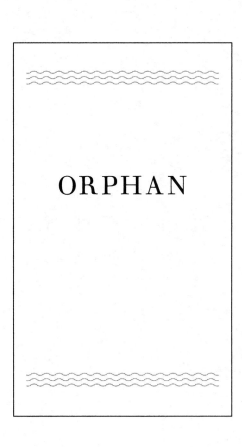

ORPHAN

DURING MY FIRST MONTH AS WARD RESIDENT, I was assigned to the oncology service. I hated it. Any service on which patients routinely die during morning rounds upsets me. And there were always too many patients, most of them being treated for some terminal process with drugs that made them sick to just this side of death and not infrequently beyond. Some doctors enjoy this kind of challenge; I'm not one of them. It scared me. I was twenty years older than the rest of the residents in the hospital, and it shook me in some way I wasn't able even to name. As if some vulnerability within me were waiting to declare itself. Something that, like cancer, I would discover only after it was too late.

Which may have been why, that month at least, I tended to leave the routine business of the service to my competent intern, Mike, and on the weekends didn't mind looking after my orphan. "Orphan" is the name given to any intern admitting patients when her own resident isn't around; on weekends when I was admitting, one of my responsibilities was to supervise the orphan also admitting that day.

The current orphan's name was Virginia; she went by Virgie, and she was assigned to the gastrointestinal, or GI, service. This is another subspecialty the house staff tends to regard with distaste, but compared to oncology it seemed to me a clean, well-lighted place. True, the patients include a fair number of GI bleeders, who require close watching but never quite buy the transfer to, say, a surgical bed that would get them off your census. You usually also have two or three patients in the final stages of liver failure, who are generally delirious, capable of taking sudden nasty turns, and infected with viruses you don't want to bring home to your family. Add to that the pancreatitis patients (unstable alcoholics who withdraw under your care), the inflammatory bowel patients (unhappy), and the occasional fecal impaction (don't ask), and you can understand why, when Virgie returned my page that morning, she sounded a little harried.

"Just checking in," I said. "How's your day going?"

"It's horrible," she cried. "We just finished rounding and I've got three discharges to get out and a float down in the ER I haven't even seen yet."

As problems go, I thought, this wasn't bad. Discharges were a good thing. And the patient in the ER was probably stable. But for the sake of form I asked.

"I think so," Virgie said. "Some bogus abdominal pain thing. But I don't know when I'm going to see her. Could you go? I'll get there as soon as I can."

"Take your time," I said soothingly. "Happy to help out."

"Thank you thank you thank you," she cried, and hung up.

I was happy, I realized as I made my way down the quiet back stairs to the basement. Somebody else's patient to see. Already worked up. Probably not dying. More of a social visit than anything else.

Ten-thirty on a Saturday morning, and the emergency department was already busy. Most of the bays were occupied, and the noise was enough to make ordinary conversation difficult; there were shouts coming from one of the trauma bays on my right. I ran my eye over the bank of monitors suspended above the front desk, checking the list of patients for anything that looked like it might be coming my way. The one good thing about oncology was that it tended to get its admissions from clinic, and the clinic wasn't open on weekends. But sicklers, intractable pain, clotting problems of various sorts, and the occasional blast crisis could come in at any time. And once the other services filled up, we would be in line for whatever needed admitting. But the board seemed clear for now, so I looked for the name Virgie had given me. I found her on the first screen, Bay 7: *Crawley, A.*, her name in pink to indicate her sex. Her time of arrival the night before (10:42) was highlighted in orange, a token of the emergency department's outrage at her continued presence here. This probably accounted for some of Virginia's urgency about her pending discharges: she was undoubtedly getting pressure from bed control to free up space for incoming admissions.

I pulled the chart for Bay 7. This is a bed at the front of the ER, where they like to keep the unstable ones. I wasn't sure what there was about Crawley that merited this. I registered this question, like most questions in the hospital, as a pang, a surge of doubt that distracted me as I thumbed through the untidy stack of papers on the clipboard.

A. Crawley was a float—a patient worked up by the night shift and handed over to an intern the next morning for ongoing care. Floats are notoriously iffy: the system has too many cracks where orders, lab results, sometimes entire patients can get lost; and the workup, conducted by a resident whose internal clock is even more messed up than usual, can vary from merely sketchy to outright delusional. It had been drummed into me early in my training: always eyeball the float.

The admission note told me little. This was a twenty-two-year-old female who had come in with a one-day history of nausea, vomiting, and abdominal pain. No significant medical history, no drug allergies, no sick exposures except to a dog known (how, I could not begin to guess) to harbor parvovirus B19. It was clear this was a red herring included in the history in a display of mere thoroughness: factual, obscure, irrelevant. Ms. Crawley had endured her nausea, vomiting, and abdominal pain for approximately twelve hours, at which point she had attempted to treat it with a few Tylenol Sinus tablets. When those failed to bring relief, she came in to the ED.

As stories went, it sounded odd. Twelve hours of a bellyache don't usually bring otherwise healthy young people to the hospital. I was left with a familiar mix of annoyance (this was wasting my time), relief (nothing horrible was going to happen), and dread (what was I missing?). According to this script, the lady shouldn't have come in. But she had. And they'd put her up front in Bay 7 where they could keep an eye on her. Why?

I scanned the rest of the note. The review of systems—that laundry list of symptoms with which we catechize admissions ("Anyfeverschillsnightsweatsweightlosschestpaincoughor changeinthecolorofyourstools?")—added nothing to the history. Physical exam ditto: mild abdominal tenderness. Meaningless. The labs and X-rays seemed to rule out any specifically abdominal pathology. But there were two false notes that got my attention. Her white count was slightly elevated, indicating a possible infection. And her serum lactate was high. This was the one that made me stop and look up for a moment.

An elevated lactate accompanied by a high white count explained why they had lodged her in the front of the ED rather than stashing her in the back room with the sore throats and bladder infections. Lactic acid is a by-product of cellular metabolism gone astray. In company with a high white count, it signals sepsis: infection at large in the circulation, and a patient hours away from the ICU.

None of which fit the innocuous history of A. Crawley.

I scanned the admission note again, wondering if there was anything I'd overlooked. But there was nothing there; the only other lab value remotely notable was the serum Tylenol level. We check Tylenol levels pretty frequently: it's at once an extremely common and potentially a very nasty drug. Toxicity can occur at less then twice the recommended dose. And when somebody, in a suicidal gesture or simple confusion, downs an entire bottle, there isn't much time to get help. If the antidote isn't started within twelve hours of ingestion, the patient is basically dead (although the dying can go on for weeks). But given Crawley's history and the time they had drawn the sample, the level they had gotten wasn't worrying: it was consistent with a reasonable dose taken at the time she had reported, about four or five hours before she came to the ER. But they had thought to check: that was interesting.

The history didn't do much for me except to rouse vague fears of doom—and what day in the hospital doesn't do that? Abdominal pain and infection: the possible causes of such a pairing make a long list, and some of them can be serious trouble. Fortunately for my orphan, the common ones—appendicitis, gallbladder disease—are surgical issues. And until A. Crawley developed signs or symptoms of needing transfer to surgery, there wasn't much for Virgie to do. Time would tell. We would watch her, and wait (as the saying goes) for her to declare.

That should have been all. But I thought again about the Tylenol, and I saw that the ED had been thinking about it too. They had started her on N-acetylcysteine, the specific antidote for Tylenol, around six a.m. Her levels didn't warrant it, but it's an innocuous drug (except for the taste), so I could see their logic. Not knowing what to treat, they had treated what they could.

When I look back at those years in the hospital, I can see that this kind of nervous second-guessing might seem, to anyone on the outside, hysterical. At the time, however, for me and I think for most of the house staff, it was simply a way of life. During those years, I always felt that I knew nothing. And no matter how much you did know, there was always more you didn't. In that vast desert of ignorance always lurked that one detail waiting to kill somebody. Which was bad enough if you were prone to worrying about such things. What made it worse was that you were required—by the patient, the family, the intern—to look as if you knew what you were doing. You couldn't turn and ask someone else. And you couldn't count on second chances. I'd learned that years before.

So it must have been an irrationally optimistic impulse that made me look around again, hoping to find somebody who could tell me anything else about A. Crawley. But there was nobody. The nurse said only, "She's a flake. When are you going to get her out of here?"

I knocked on the door, pausing briefly before pushing through. The room was dim. The bed occupied the back half. Curled up in it was a slender, pretty young woman under a cotton ER blanket and a tangle of sheets. She wore a hospital gown. The inevitable bag of saline hung over her, dripping through an angiocath taped to her left forearm. In the far corner, the usual pile of clothing, shoes, and purse lay heaped on a chair. The patient was already awake, watching me. In the corner behind the door, a long male figure sprawled half out of a chair, stirring as I entered.

I introduced myself. A. Crawley stretched carefully, propped herself up on one elbow, and took my offered hand. She didn't look too sick.

"I hope you won't think I'm bad," she drawled. She said this with a sly half smile, waiting for a reaction.

It was such an odd thing to say that I paused.

"Why would I think that?"

She shrugged, still smiling. "I don't know." And slowly she slid back down to the bed. She was still looking at me.

The oddness of her opening gambit hovered in the room. I didn't know what to do with it, so I set it aside, plunging into the ritual. How did she feel? Not so good: her stomach hurt. When did that start? This morning—no, it's yesterday now, isn't it. She stopped with a giggle, and a girlish movement of the shoulders that made her seem ten years younger than she was, until she caught it with a sudden intake of breath. My thoughts went haring after the abdominal pathologies that might make it painful to move like that. It's not a short list.

We plowed on through, and I heard the same story I'd gotten from the admission note, minus the irrelevant dog. The repetition of the history should have been reassuring, but—oddly—it was not. I had been waiting for an inconsistency, something that might account for the strange atmosphere in the room, the opaqueness of her chart—waiting for anything, preferably something psychiatric and therefore harmless. But she wasn't a nut. Her story was lucid, at least. And yet the strange atmosphere persisted. She giggled at odd moments, went shy at others, and generally carried on like a naughty teen. Something was off here, but I couldn't figure it. She was a flake, I told myself. Her belly hurt. Watch her declare. I let the exam cement the story: a healthy young woman with normal active bowel sounds, slightly tender in the epigastric region.

Virgie came in, filling up the rest of the space in the room with her own awkwardness and hurry. I made the introductions, Virgie performed a perfunctory exam, and we excused ourselves.

Out in the ED it was getting on toward noon, and the noise level had gone up a notch; the hollering from the trauma bays had died down, but from everywhere else came the clamor of people speaking: words laid on words until they formed a resisting medium, a substance you could almost feel parting as you passed through. We retreated behind the counter and lodged against the cubbies, where I reshelved the clipboard.

"You've got to scan her belly," I shouted over the din.

"Why?" Virgie spoke petulantly, out of the intern's settled resistance to adding anything.

"Belly pain, white count. You've got to. And did you see her lactate?"

Virgie flustered. "She's got a lactate?"

Then to cover her omission she started asking me all the questions you run through to find the cause of an elevated lactate. I knew the questions too. I just didn't know the answers.

"You need to scan her belly," I repeated. "Get it started down here." I flipped through the papers on the board. "She's written for a floor bed. She should probably be in step-down, but the floor is all we're going to get."

"I can write her for frequent vitals."

"Do that." I handed her the clipboard. "But it's no substitute for step-down, you know."

"I'll keep an eye on her," she muttered as she scribbled orders.

I watched her, her hair astray, white coat grubby, clutching her pen between her teeth as she reached up to grab a new order sheet. There was a slightly wild look about her, an extra millimeter or so of white showing around her irises. The odds of Virgie finding time to keep an eye on A. Crawley struck me as pretty slim.

CT-abdomen-pelvis-w/contrast, she wrote out. *Abd pain &* ↑ *wbc/lactate.*

"Make it stat," I added as an afterthought. "And tell her nurse."

Despite what you may see doctors do on TV, I hardly ever order anything stat. You can get a bad reputation. Everyone knows that what you really mean is, *I forgot to order this and I want to go home for dinner.* Today it meant something else. Vague fears. Impending doom. *Abd pain &* ↑ *wbc/lactate.*

AROUND FOUR THAT AFTERNOON, Mike, my intern, paged me with the news that we had two new admissions waiting in the ER: a young man with sickle-cell disease and joint pain and a chemotherapy patient who had been vomiting uncontrollably for several days. I told him to start on the sickler; sickle-cell pain crises are usually routine, and beyond the need to make sure the patient's marrow and lungs are still working, management is a matter of ordering IV fluids, narcotics, and the laxative of choice. I went to the nearest workstation to look up the records of the other patient, a young woman with metastatic breast cancer and a recent history of frequent admissions for nausea and vomiting. She had three young children and seemed to do better when someone took care of her for a change. We'd treat her and send her home, she'd take care of her children until she needed to come in again, and it was going to go on like that until one day she wouldn't go home. Armoring myself dully against the implications of this, I lumbered down to the ER to talk to her, trying not to think about anything but the treatment of nausea.

I SHOVED THE CLIPBOARD for Bay 11 back into its slot and fished a blank order sheet off the top shelf. The shelf is a bit of a reach for me, and as I stood there, stretched high on tiptoe, I found myself staring at a pair of surgery residents a few feet away. I knew the senior, Sara Barnes, a fifth-year unusual among her kind for a helpful civility with the other house staff. She was in earnest conversation with her intern, a sour-faced young woman who looked ready to quit. They were holding a large dark square of radiography print up to the overhead fluorescents. I recognized the patchwork of a CT scan. Sara gestured to a series of images on the lower third of the print.

"There," she was saying. "See it? Where the contrast makes that little V and stops?"

"Yeah," said the intern.

Sara ignored her tone. "It's classic. They call it arrowhead sign: it's practically pathognomonic for appendicitis."

"Okay," said the intern.

Appendicitis is, by definition, a surgical emergency. I'd actually seen it only twice in my life, during rotations in medical school. As my hand groped along a seemingly empty shelf, I found myself automatically rehearsing what I knew about appendicitis. That little worm at the base of the colon gets blocked off for any number of reasons; infection, inflammation, and swelling set in, along with nausea, and pain so variable in its location as to be notoriously misleading; pretty soon the organ gets so distended it cuts off its own blood supply. Tissue dies.

And as it dies, it produces lactate.

"We've got to find whoever ordered this," Sara said, and her eyes started questing around the room.

My hand by this time had found the order sheet it was looking for, but I was no longer concerned with what my hand had found.

"Is that Crawley?" I called. "Is that Ariel Crawley's CT? I ordered that."

It took Sara a moment to focus on me. Then the two of them were around me, barking.

I let them go on, cherishing the growing warmth of my realization that they were talking about taking A. Crawley to the OR tonight. Even though this would ultimately benefit Virgie, not me, I couldn't help but feel a flush of misplaced pride. Virgie would emerge from her call night with one fewer patient to round on in the morning. Good for Virgie. I was taking care of my orphan.

Sara and her intern left, busy, satisfied. I placed a page to Virgie to let her know. And then I sat down to order ondansetron and Ativan for the patient I'd just admitted in 11, whom

I could still see, through a gap in the curtains, retching in a basin, a mauve turban askew on her hairless skull.

AROUND EIGHT P.M. I was up on 3 Central, passing through on my way from the ED, where our last two admissions of the day were still having the finishing touches added to their admission orders. I was on my way up to the cancer ward, where the patient in the turban was still vomiting. There was little purpose in my putting in an appearance, having ordered more Ativan for her over the phone, but I felt the obligation. And the ER was making me weary. While admitting our full five patients, I had also helped Virgie with three more. She still had two scheduled transfers, both end-stage livers for transplant evaluation, coming in by plane from elsewhere, and both delayed by weather. I had no idea what weather might be happening outside to delay the air ambulance, but I was glad of it. My own intern had capped. We had survived. All that remained for me to do was to help Mike get his patients settled. Then I could scuttle off to my call room and try to sleep.

I ducked into the 3 Central nursing station and called up Virgie's census. A. Crawley should be on her way off it, heading to surgery. But you can't take things like that for granted in the hospital, which is why transfers are dangerous; sometimes people fall into the cracks. I needed to check.

She was still on Virgie's census, lodged inevitably in one of the rooms far down the hallway, at the end of a cul-de-sac.

The back corner of 3 Central was not a good place to be. There was an old story in circulation about a patient on that hallway dialing 911: the nurse had ignored her call bell that long. The story was almost certainly apocryphal, but like most hospital legends it reflected a truth. The biggest threat to Ariel Crawley, stuck back in that corner with her gangrenous appendix, was that between scheduled vital signs no one would simply happen to walk by. I wondered when Virgie had last looked in on her, and as I clicked through the workstation to get at labs, I paged Virgie.

Crawley's seven p.m. labs were coming up on the screen just as the telephone rang.

"Virgie," I said. She said something very fast and incoherent in return.

Or maybe it was me. Certainly my own thoughts went suddenly too fast to follow as numbers outlined in red seemed to fill up the screen.

"I just got a page from Core Labs," Virgie was saying. I was forcing my eyes to attend to the numbers, forcing them to make sense. Two of Crawley's liver chemistries, her AST and ALT, were over ten thousand. The normal values are less than fifty.

"Her LFTs?" I said. "I'm looking at them right now."

There was panic in Virgie's voice. "What's going on?"

The liver—that dense, strongly flavored organ that occupies the right upper quadrant of the belly—does a great many things, most of which I could not recall at that moment beyond a distinct sense that they were essential to life. The transaminases, AST and ALT, are chemicals the liver produces for use in its inscrutable tasks. When the liver is damaged, they leak into the blood. What A. Crawley was demonstrating, as her transaminases jumped from essentially normal levels on arrival at the ED the night before to these sky-high values now, was fulminant liver failure.

I scanned the other chemistries, but nothing else was out of line—yet: by morning, other numbers would start to waver and slide into the red; the bilirubin the liver is supposed to clear from the blood would wind up circulating instead, tinting her eyes a muddy yellow; the coagulation factors the liver produces would start to fail, and she would begin to bleed. Then she would slip into a coma. And not long after that she would die.

And in a flash I knew what was doing it, as certainly as I knew where it would end. The appendicitis was a distraction, irrelevant to the real issue. I knew what had destroyed her liver. I knew it as surely as I knew that, for all practical purposes, A. Crawley was already dead.

I STOOD UP INVOLUNTARILY, impelled by adrenaline. I had no purpose in mind, no notion of anything I could do to change the course of things. It was too late to help A. Crawley; in a jumble of ugly images I imagined what her next few days would be like. Just what I wanted as I stalked toward her room, I had no idea: I wasn't trying to do anything, or to learn anything as banal as why. I think I just needed to see her.

The door at the end of the hall was ajar, light visible through the opening. I knocked once and went through. The bed in that room is wedged across the far end, the rest of the room a long architectural afterthought. She was awake, her bedding disheveled, the expression on her face inscrutable as she watched me traverse the floor. The boyfriend was not in evidence. The visitor chair was occupied by a well-dressed older woman I took for the mother. With a cursory nod at her, I knelt at the bedside.

"Ms. Crawley," I said. I tried to sound calm.

"Hi," she said. She did not giggle, but a smile flirted across her face, turning down at the end.

"How are you feeling?"

"Terrible. Those horrible doctors."

"What doctors?" I remembered Sara Barnes and her intern. I wondered what they had said to her. If they had seen the labs yet.

The pout became a look of frank distaste. "The surgeons."

I glanced at her mussed bedclothes and suppressed a smile. The surgical abdominal exam. "Mash on you pretty hard?"

"I thought they were going to cut me right here." She attempted the smile again.

"Did they tell you—" I began, then stopped.

"Do I really need an operation?"

She looked puzzled, like someone who has been told out of the blue she needs surgery. Nothing more.

I could feel at my back the mother shifting in her chair. I glanced at her. She was leaning forward, worried: her daughter needed an operation.

"Ma'am?" I said finally. The mother cocked her head.

"Would you mind excusing us for a moment? I'd like to talk to your daughter."

The mother, now more worried but that couldn't be helped, told her daughter she'd be right back, gathered up a large leather purse, and softly closed the door behind her.

I turned back to the patient.

"Ms. Crawley," I said.

"Yes?" Still—unaccountably, maddeningly—a little coy.

"What did you do?"

The smile faded. Her eyes went elsewhere.

"You know what I'm talking about."

"No." She would not look up.

"When did you take it?"

No answer.

"It wasn't last night, was it?"

No answer.

"When did you take it, Ariel?" I never first-name my patients. But I called her Ariel, and I wasn't sure if I was pleading or threatening.

Her hand made an angry shoving gesture, pushing a wrinkle across the sheet.

"Ariel, if you don't tell me, you're going to die. Do you understand that? You're going to die. If you want any chance of living past the next three days, you have to tell me what you did."

As if it matters, I said to myself, in that cynical inner voice that kept me company throughout my residency. But certainly it sounded like it mattered. I realized I was on the verge of shouting. I was shaking with something, some sensation so close to me I couldn't identify it.

Did I really care? It is in the nature of the house staff to become uncaring (even though, in the hospital, not to care is to be brutal). There is so much death and suffering and grief, and in the midst of it we still need to fill out forms, subject the sick to indignities and pain, try to eat and sleep and keep all these needy people at some kind of distance. When I wasn't too numb, I worried that I'd stopped caring.

And now I was berating a dying woman because she wouldn't tell me exactly what she'd done. Maybe I had too many feelings. Or none at all.

She didn't speak, but she stopped the restless motions of her hands and held still on the bed. I was still as well, and for a long moment neither one of us moved.

"I'm hurting," she said finally.

Another silence, a vast empty space.

"Where?"

"In here." She gestured at her abdomen. And then her eyes turned up to meet mine. "Is that what it does?"

I nodded. She dropped her gaze back to the bedsheet, the fingers of her left hand spread over the fabric. A tear fell from her cheek to spot the linen beside her thumb. "I didn't know," she said.

Didn't know what? I wanted to ask, but there were more pressing questions, and I never found out what she didn't know.

Instead I made her tell me how much Tylenol she had taken. Maybe thirty, maybe forty. She didn't count. And not the night before. She'd said last night when they'd asked her, but it was Thursday she meant. Thursday night. Her voice was small, emotionless, tired. She had let her secret out, and it was much too late to matter. I think she knew that without being told.

But I had to tell her anyway. I quietly explained to her the difference that day made. It felt much more brutal than shouting. The Tylenol level they had drawn in the ER was just a number. By itself, the number was meaningless. To interpret it, you had to know how much time had elapsed between the taking of the drug and the drawing of the blood. If it had been a matter of a few hours, her level was fine and all was well. If it had been more like thirty hours, then the number they drew was the tail end of a massive overdose.

And perhaps the worst of it was that it didn't matter: her lie, her silence, made no difference to the story. It wouldn't have mattered if she had confessed right away. She had come to the hospital too late. The antidote the ED had given, out of its characteristic pessimism, hadn't been able to help her. Nothing could. The only difference her lie made was to something far outside the realm of medicine.

I knelt there beside her while she sniffled quietly and her shoulders shook.

I'd like to say that I held her, or said soothing words. But I don't hold female patients, even when they cry, and I had no soothing words. I knelt there and watched her, and struggled to comprehend what I saw.

Ariel was suspended, here, in this room with me, between life and death. Her liver had failed. She would surely die. But just now, and for a while longer, she would lie here on her bed, her belly sore where Sara Barnes had poked it, and cry. She was alive and she was dead, somehow occupying both states at once until the passage of time would collapse them into one. And I knelt at her bed in some paralysis of awe, powerless and hollow at the core.

I HAD FELT THAT sensation once before. Long before I went into medicine, back when I still had hopes of making a living as a writer, my wife and I were invited to a dinner party one oppressively hot Saturday in July. Our host, a pleasant Swiss who taught German at my wife's college, had prepared a meal of broiled fish preceded by a delicate, steaming soup— the kind of meal only a foreigner would think of preparing on a scorching Summer day. But he was proud of it, and we had the sense to appreciate his cooking, and praised especially the soup, which was the least dense of the evening's offerings, even if it steamed.

"Wild mushrooms," he said, explaining the subtle flavor of the broth. "My mother gathered them herself in the Alps."

"Ah," we said, and sipped the soup.

That night around two a.m. we both awoke, sharp pains in our bellies and a strange hollow sensation. "The soup," we said at once, aghast at the possibility even while we laughed and dismissed it, lying down again to sleep. But sleep would not come. By half past two it was clear that something bad was going on, and ten minutes later it was equally clear that we could no longer laugh away the one idea that had seized our imaginations from the moment we had voiced it. I rose from bed to look up the number for poison control.

The voice at the other end of the line was professionally calm, faultlessly polite. After a brief discussion of our symptoms and the meal that had preceded them, the woman said to me, "It certainly does sound like the mushrooms. Unfortunately, if that's the case, there's very little that can be done: from the symptoms you describe, I'm afraid it's too late to do anything." A brief silence on the line, and then she spoke again. "But before you go to the hospital, you must call your host. He'll need to contact anyone else who had the soup."

I hung up the phone. I understand now that what the voice on the other end of the line had meant by "too late" was simply "it will have to run its course." That the course could end in our deaths was another part of what she hadn't said, but there are many kinds of mushrooms, and not all of them are deadly. At the time, I didn't know that.

I let my hand lie on the receiver while a minute passed. My hand looked as if it were something somebody had left there. It was three in the morning on a sullen July night. Out the kitchen window I could see the full moon floating in a brown sky. In a moment I would move again. In a moment I would go back down the hall and tell my wife what I had heard. In a moment.

I stood there for what seemed a long time, hearing nothing of the night noises, only a dull roaring in my ears, while I put off the moment when I would move and time would begin again.

I pulled my hand from the telephone and walked back through the darkened house, stopping at the door of what was going to be the baby's room. It still smelled of fresh paint. I stood there a moment and thought, So this is how it feels.

That was all I could come up with: This is how it feels to be dead. I stood at the door of the empty room for a long time, feeling nothing.

We were not, of course, dead. Hans had been joking about his mother gathering mushrooms. He had bought them at the Pathmark that afternoon. He was somewhat testy about this, a little too annoyed with the three a.m. phone call to be properly remorseful (I felt) about the spoiled fish he had served us after the soup. My wife and I endured nothing worse than three days of nausea, a week of depressed appetite, and an aversion to mushrooms that lingers to this day.

Nothing worse than that.

As for Ariel Crawley, after she told me the time of her overdose, she begged me not to tell her mother. *Why not?* I wanted to ask, but I restrained myself. It was of a piece with whatever hurt she had been trying to treat with Tylenol. And it no longer mattered. I told her that her medical condition was nobody's business but her own, and that the hospital would respect her privacy. It was up to her to tell her mother as much or as little as she chose. Then I left the room.

I left under some sense of urgency, feeling there were things I should do. But other than placing a few phone calls, there wasn't anything, really. The ED had already ordered the antidote, and it was clear that it wasn't working. I let Virginia know what I had learned, and called the ICU to let them know they could be getting a transfer before the night was over. Then I remembered Sara Barnes, and called her as well. She was puzzled by the information, liver failure and Tylenol toxicity not fitting into her protocols any more than appendicitis fit into mine, but she concluded that it didn't change anything. The patient's appendix was still a surgical emergency; her attending was on his way in; Ariel Crawley was posted for the OR that evening. As for her liver, after a word or two about involving Hepatology post-op the conversation slid off into silence.

IT DIDN'T END THERE. Ariel Crawley fell off my radar later that evening as she was wheeled off to surgery. Her mother, looking no more concerned than any woman would following her daughter to an emergency appendectomy, followed down the hallway with an armful of Ariel's belongings. I went home the next afternoon, hearing nothing more until several days later, when I learned that she had had her appendix successfully removed before midnight Saturday. And that two days later she had undergone a successful liver transplant. Her youth, her fundamental health, the abruptness of her failure, had all catapulted her to the head of the list, and through another stroke of luck a suitable donor came in, the helmetless passenger of a wrecked motorcycle, and now she was in the surgical ICU, holding her own.

Over the next several months I continued to hear of Ariel's progress. There were the usual post-transplant problems, but the last I heard she was doing as well as can be expected. Life with someone else's liver is never easy: episodes of rejection, toxicities of immune-suppressing drugs, the threat of infection. But I lost eight patients that month, and Ariel wasn't one of them. She got a second chance. A victory of sorts.

I know I'm not really entitled to claim any kind of victory here: my contribution, in the end, was to order a CT that bought her an irrelevant surgery, and to force a confession, too late, to something that was obvious anyway. But I'll claim my victories where I can, earned or not.

Did Ariel deserve hers? The question lingers, but I have no answers. Ariel's out there somewhere, I hope, living her life somehow, while others sicken and die waiting for transplants that never come. Maybe no one earns a second chance. Who would be worthy of it? But we did have a baby, and even (God blessed us) another. I started writing again. Residency passed like a bad dream, and on awaking I found I cared again. Perhaps too much.

All victories are worth claiming, when we consider the alternatives. And when we recognize that all such victories are temporary, forestalling that dead moment in the middle of the night.

THE
PERFECT
CODE

A FAINT CLICK OPENS THE AIR. A DISEMBODIED voice calls out, "Adult Code 100, Adult Code 100, 5 East. Adult Code 100, 5 East." Or it might be "Code Blue, Code Blue 3C, Code Blue 3C." From place to place the wording varies, but the message thinly hidden in the code is always the same: somewhere in the hospital, someone is dying.

The nature of the emergency varies as well. Hearts stop. Vital signs droop. We give up the ghost. But whatever the nature of the emergency, the response is the same: from all over the hospital the code team comes running, and the attempt at resuscitation begins.

The team is an invention of the 1960s, when evidence began to suggest that people suffering cardiopulmonary arrest had a much better chance of surviving if organized help reached them within two minutes. The "code" part was a response to public relations concerns that the laity might be upset by announcements of "Cardiac arrest on 4 North." Hence the "Code"—100, blue, pick your meaningless term. Thanks to television, I doubt anyone is taken in by it these days. But it adds another element of insider status to a culture that values that sort of thing.

Despite being no secret to anyone, the code still holds its mysteries. I'm not sure, still, just what I have learned by running to so many codes. But the experience haunts me, long after the fact. As if, somewhere in the tangle of tubes and wires, knotted sheets, Betadine, and blood, I lost track of something important. Listen.

IN THE HOSPITAL WHERE I work, codes go something like this. A nurse finds a patient slumped over in bed. The nurse calls her name. No answer. The nurse shakes her. No answer. Harder. Still no answer. The nurse steps to the door and calls, in tones that rise at each syllable, "I need some help here." The rest of the nurses on the floor converge. Within a minute, every bystander within hearing is gathered at the door.

In the basement of the hospital, a hospital operator listens intently to her headset. She flips a switch, and a faint click opens the hospital to the microphone on her console. "Adult Code 100, 6 South. Adult Code 100, 6 South." The message goes out on the hospital PA system, her bodiless voice filling the hallways. It also goes out to a system of antique voice pagers, from which the operator's measured words emerge as inarticulate squealing. The pagers are largely backup, in case some member of the team is, say, in the bathroom, or otherwise out of reach of the PA system.

The team consists of eight or nine people: respiratory techs,

anesthesiologists, pharmacists, and the residents on call for
the cardiac ICU. On hearing the summons, the residents drop
whatever they are doing and sprint. People running full-tilt
in a hospital is unavoidably a spectacle. In their voluminous
white coats, from whose pockets fall stethoscopes, penlights,
reflex hammers, EKG calipers, tuning forks, ballpoint pens
(these clatter across the floors, to be scooped up by the medical
student who follows behind), the medical team's passing is a
curious combination of high drama and burlesque.

The medical team arrives on a scene of Bedlam. The room
is so crowded with nurses, CNAs, janitors, and miscellaneous
onlookers that it can be physically impossible to enter. Shoul-
dering your way through the mob at the door, you are stopped
by a crowd around the bed; the crash cart, a rolling red metal
Sears Roebuck toolchest, is also in the way, its open drawers a
menace to knees and elbows. There are wires draped from the
crash cart, and tubing everywhere.

At the center of all this lies the patient, the only one in the
room who isn't shouting. She doesn't move at all. This time it
is an elderly woman, frail to the point of wasting; her ribs arch
above her hollow belly. Her eyes are half open, her jaw is slack,
pink tongue protruding slightly. Her gown and the bedding
are tangled in a mass at the foot of the bed; at a glance you take
in the old mastectomy scar, the scaphoid abdomen, the gray
tuft between her legs. At the head of the bed, a nurse is pressing a mask over her face, squeezing oxygen through a large
bag; the woman's cheeks puff out with each squeeze, which
isn't right. Another nurse is compressing the chest, not hard
enough. You shoulder her aside and press two fingers under

the angle of the jaw. Nothing. A quick listen at her chest: only the hubbub in the room, dulled by silent flesh. Pile the heels of both hands over her breastbone and start to push: the bed rolls away. Falling half onto the patient, you holler above the commotion, "Somebody please lock the bed." Alternate this with, "Does anyone have the chart?"

A nurse near the door hoists a thick brown binder, passing it over the heads jamming the room. "Code status," you bawl out. "Full code," the nurse bawls back. You reposition your hands and push down on her breastbone. "Why's she here?" There is a palpable crunch as her ribs separate from her sternum. "Metastatic breast cancer," the nurse calls, flipping pages in the chart. "Admitted for pain control." You lighten up the pressure and continue to push, rhythmically, fast. You look around, trying to pick out from the mass of excited bystanders the people who belong; the background is a weird frieze of faces and limbs reaching, pointing, gesticulating, mouths open. The noise is immense. On the opposite side of the bed you see one of the respiratory techs has arrived. "Airway," you shout, and the tech nods: she has already seen the puffing cheeks. She takes the mask and bag from the nurse and adjusts the patient's neck. The patient's chest starts to rise and fall beneath your hands.

"What's she getting for pain?"

"Morphine PCA."

"What rate?"

The question sets off a flurry of activity among some nurses, one of whom stoops to examine the IV pump at the patient's bedside. "Two per hour, one q fifteen on the lockout."

"Narcan," you order.

By this time the pharmacist has arrived, which is fortunate because you can't remember the dose of opiate-blocker. You doubt this is overdose here, but it's the first thing to try. Out of the corner of your eye you see the pharmacist load a clear ampule into a syringe and pass it to a nurse.

Meanwhile, on your left, the other resident and the intern are plunging large needles into both groins, probing for the femoral vein. The intern strikes blood first, removes the syringe, throws it onto the sheets. "Send that off for labs," you shout. Blood dribbles from the needle's hub as the intern threads a long, coiled wire through it into the vein. The other resident stops jabbing and watches the intern's progress. With a free hand she feels for the femoral pulse, but the bed is bouncing. You stop compressing. The resident focuses, shakes her head. Start compressing again.

A nurse reaches around you on the right, trying to fit a pair of metallic adhesive pads onto the patient's chest. You shake your head. "Paddles," you shout. "Get me the paddles." Then, into the general roar, "Somebody take that syringe and send it off for labs." A hand grabs the syringe and whisks it off. "You," you shout at the med student, who is hanging by the resident's elbow. "Get a gas." The resident throws a package from the crash cart, then steps back to give the student access to the patient's groin. The student fits the needle—it's a sixteen-guage, two inches long—to the blood gas syringe, feels for the pulse your compressions are making in the groin, and stabs it home: blood, dark purple, fills the barrel. The student looks worried; he may have missed the artery. It doesn't matter. The student passes it around the foot of the bed to another hand and it vanishes.

The nurse at your elbow is still there, holding the defibrillator paddles. She stands as though she has been holding these out to you for some time. Clap the paddles on the patient's chest. Over your shoulder on the tiny screen of the defibrillator a wavy line of green light scrawls horizontally onward. You look back at the other resident. "Anything?" you both say at once, and both of you shake your heads. The intern has finished with the femoral catheter, very fast. He holds up one of the access ports. "Amp of epi," you say, but there's no response. Louder: "I need an amp of epi." Finally someone shoves a big blunt-nosed syringe into your hand. Without stopping to verify that it's what you asked for, you lean over and fit it to the port and push the plunger. Another look at the screen. Still nothing. "Atropine," you call out, and this time a nurse has it ready. "Push it," you say, and she does. Stop compressions, check the screen.

Suddenly the wavery tracing leaps into life, a jagged irregular line, teeth of a painful saw. "V fib," the other resident calls out, annoying you for a moment. You clamp the paddles down on the patient's ribs. "Everyone clear?" Everyone has moved back two feet from the bed. You check your own legs, arch your back: "Clear?" You push the button. The patient spasms, then lies limp again. The pattern on the screen is unchanged. The other resident shakes her head. You call over your shoulder, "Three hundred," and shock again. The body twitches again. An unpleasant smell rises from the bed.

The pattern on the screen subsides, back to the long lazy

wave. Still no pulse. You start compressing again. "Epi," you call out. "Atropine." There is another flutter of activity on the screen, but before you can shock, it goes flat again, almost flat, perhaps there is a suggestion of a ragged rhythm there, fine sawteeth. "Clear," you call again, and everybody draws back. "Three-sixty," you remember to say over your shoulder, and when the answering call comes back you shock again, knowing this is futile. But the patient is dead and there is no harm in trying. As the body slumps again, there is a palpable slackening of the noise level in the room, and even though you go on another ten minutes, pushing on the chest until your shoulders are burning and your breath is short, and a total of ten milligrams of epinephrine have gone in, there is nothing more on the monitor that looks remotely shockable.

Finally, you straighten up, and find the clock on the wall. "I'm calling it," you say. Against the wall, a nurse with a clipboard makes a note. "Time?" she says. You tell her.

There is more. Picking up, writing notes, a phone call or two. There is a family member in the hallway, sitting stricken on a bench beside a nurse or volunteer holding a hand. You need to speak to her, but before you do you have to find out the patient's name. Or you don't. And then you go back to whatever you were doing before the code went out over the PA.

WHAT I'M THINKING, USUALLY, as we trickle out at the end, is this: What a mess.

There is a great deal of mess in hospital medicine, literal and figurative, and the code bunches it all up into a dense mass that on some days seems to represent everything wrong with the world. The haste, the turmoil, the anonymity, the smell, the futility: all of it brought to bear on a single body, the body inert at the center of the mess, as if at the center of all wrong it remains somehow inviolate, beyond help or harm; as if to point a moral I would understand better if I only had time to stop and contemplate it. Which I don't, not that day. We're admitting and there are three patients, two on the floor and one down in the ER, waiting to be seen. There is no time to read the fine print on anything, least of all the mortal contract just executed on the anonymous woman lying back in that room. I can barely make out the large block letters at the top: Our Patients Die. And very often they do so in the middle of a scene with all the dignity of a food fight in a high school cafeteria. We can't cure everybody, but I think most of us treasure as a small consolation that at least we can afford people some kind of dignity at the end, something quiet and solemn in which whatever meaning resides in all of this may be—if we watch and listen carefully—perceptible.

Which may be why one particular code persists in my memory, long after the event, as the perfect code.

DAVID GILLET WAS THE name I got from the medicine admitting officer. I wasn't sure what to make of the MAO's story, but I knew I didn't like it.

The story was an eighty-two-year-old guy with a broken neck. He had apparently fallen in his bathroom that morning, cracking his first and second vertebrae. I had a vague memory from medical school that this wasn't a good thing—the expression "hangman's fracture" kept bobbing up from the well of facts I do not use—but I had a much more distinct impression that this was not a case for cardiology.

"And Ortho isn't taking him because?" I said wearily.

"Because he's got internal organs, dude."

I sighed. "So why me?"

"Because they got an EKG."

The MAO was clearly enjoying himself. I remembered he had recently been accepted to a cardiology fellowship. I braced myself for the punch line.

"And?"

"And there's ectopy on it. *Ectopy.*" He then made a noise intended to suggest a ghost haunting something.

"Ectopy," meaning literally "out of place," refers to a heartbeat generated anywhere in the heart but the little knob in the upper right-hand corner where heartbeats are supposed to start. Such beats appear with an unusual shape and timing on the EKG. They can be caused by any number of things, from too much caffeine to fatigue to an impending heart attack, but in the absence of other warning signs ectopy is not something we generally get excited about. And it sounded to me as though a man with a broken neck had enough reasons for ectopy without sending him to the Cardiology service.

"So?" I said, trying not to sound indignant.

"So he's also got a history. Angioplasty about ten years ago, no definite history of MI. You can't really read his EKG because he's got a left bundle, no old strips so I don't know if it's new."

We were down to business.

"So I rule him out."

"You rule him out. Ortho says they'll follow with you."

"Lovely. And once I rule him out?"

"Ortho says they'll follow with you."

I said something unpleasant.

The MAO understood. "Sucks, I know, but there you are."

And there I was, down in the ER on a Sunday afternoon, turning over the stack of papers that David Gillet had generated over his six hours in the ED. There was a sheaf of EKGs covered with bizarre ectopic beats, through which occasionally emerged a stretch of normal sinus rhythm, enough to see that there was, indeed, a left bundle branch block, and not much else. The heart has several bundles, cables in its internal wiring. When some disease process disrupts a bundle, the result is an EKG too distorted to answer the question we usually ask it: Is this patient having a heart attack? Of course, the bundle itself is not a reassuring sign, and if new it merits an investigation, but plenty of people in their eighties have them and it's pretty much a so-what. But the ectopy on today's strips was impressive—if you didn't know what you were looking at you might think he was suffering some catastrophic event. I read between the lines of the consult note the orthopedic surgeons had left, and it was clear they regarded David Gillet as a time bomb, and didn't want him on their service.

Which I couldn't help noting was exactly how I felt about having a patient with a broken neck on my service. But I didn't get to make decisions like that. Instead I wadded the stack of papers back in their cubby and took a brief glance through the curtains of Bay 12. From my somewhat distorted perspective, most of what I saw of the patient was his feet, which were large, bare, and protruding from the lower end of his ER blankets in a way that suggested he would be tall if I could stand him up. At his side sat a small, iron-haired woman who at that moment was speaking to him, leaning close while she spoke. She wore a faint, affectionate smile on a face that looked otherwise tired. I watched her for a moment, her profile held precisely perpendicular to my line of sight as though posed. For a moment her face took on an almost luminous clarity, the single real object in the pallid blur of the ED, a study in patience, in care—and then it wavered, receding into a small tired woman with gray hair beside a gurney in Bay 12. The patient's face was obscured by the pink plastic horse collar that immobilized his neck. I watched the woman for a minute. Her expression, the calm progress of their conversation, suggested that nothing too drastic was going on. I took a walk to the radiology reading room to get a look at the neck films.

There were many of these, too. They showed the vulture-neck silhouette all C-spine films share. There were several unusual views, including one that I decided must have been shot straight down the patient's open mouth: it showed, framed by teeth palisaded with spiky metal, the pale ring of the first vertebra, the massive bone called the atlas, and clear (even to me) on both sides of it were two jagged dark lines angling in on the empty center where the spinal cord had failed to register on film. The break in the second vertebra was harder to make out, but I took the surgeons at their word: *C1/2 fx. Will need immobilization pending installation of halo. Will follow w/you.*

———

I WAS NOT IN the best of moods as I made my way back to the ER, grabbed a clipboard, and parted the curtains to Bay 12. I still managed an adequate smile as I introduced myself. "David Gillet?" I said tentatively.

The woman at his shoulder blinked up at me, wearing that same weary smile, brushing an iron-colored lock of hair from her face.

"It's *'Zhee-ay,'*" she said, with an odd combination of self-deprecation and something else—perhaps it was warmth?— that made me like her. "It's French," she explained. Her smile widened, one of those dazzling white things older people sometimes possess (dentures, I believe), and she welcomed me into Bay 12, which I had been inside of more times than I cared to count, with a curious air of apology, as if concerned about the quality of her housekeeping. I was charmed. This was still relatively early in the day and I was capable of being charmed. I shook myself a little, straightened my back (her posture was perfect), trying to escape some of the lethargy that had been piling on me over the day.

Her husband made a less distinct impression. The cervical stabilization collar tends to have a dampening effect on most people, as would the eight milligrams of morphine he'd absorbed over the past six hours, so it was a bleary and not very articulate history I got from him. His wife filled in the relevant bits. No prior MI. Occasional chest pain, hard to pin down (arthritis in the picture as well, of course). Otherwise a generally healthy, alert, and active man. On the one really critical point—what had caused the fall—Mr. Gillet insisted on giving account. He had *not* fainted. He had not been dizzy or breathless or experienced palpitations or anything of that sort. He had tripped. He had caught his toes on the damned bath mat, and gone down like a stupid ox. As he said the last he shook his head vehemently within the confines of his collar, and I caught my breath: you're not supposed to do that with a broken neck.

Even so I was partially reassured. The history didn't suggest a cardiac cause to his fall, and he denied any of the other symptoms that go along with impending doom. The physical exam was similarly reassuring, although hampered by the cervical collar and my dread of doing anything that might disturb his neck. He was a tall, bony man, with a nasty-looking cut across the scalp above his right eye, and dried blood crusted in his bushy eyebrows. The cut had been sutured already, and the blood made it look much worse than it was. Aside from the cut and a large bruise on his right ribs (none broken), he seemed fine. Except for the neck, of course. I stayed another few minutes, making idle chat with the wife, and then excused myself to write my orders.

HE RULED OUT WITH the four a.m. blood draw the next morning, which I announced on rounds a few hours later with less pleasure than I would have ordinarily. I knew what was coming.

"So now what?" the attending asked.

"I guess I call Ortho."

Everybody—from attending to fellow to the other resident

on the team and the intern, even the two medical students—started to smile. Then laugh.

"Well, I can call them, can't I?"

"Go ahead," the attending said.

There are attendings who will actually fight to make a transfer happen. They will call the attending on the other service and make the case, at least. Usually, when it comes to this, the transfer goes through. Which might be why most attendings are loath to let things get that far. If the patient's welfare requires it, they'll make the call (except for those dreadful individuals—and we know who they are—who believe themselves capable of caring for cases far outside their subspecialization). Or if they're dealing with some critical shortage of space. But if it's simply a matter of one patient more or less on their census, most attendings will let things be. And this attending was one of the more notoriously laissez-faire, happy enough to let the house staff run the show.

I made the call, and after three or four hours the Ortho resident returned the page. I knew by that time that I was already defeated, but I went ahead and asked the obligatory question, and received the inevitable answer (the Ortho resident having anticipated as well) that the Ortho attending did not feel comfortable taking the case—"and besides, it's not that bad a break. We'll follow."

"How long?" I asked.

"What do you mean?"

"How long does he need to be in the hospital?"

Puzzled. "When will you be done with him?"

"We've been done since eight this morning."

"You mean you'd send him home?"

"Except for the neck thing, yeah."

"Oh." This he hadn't anticipated.

"So what does he need from you?"

"He needs a halo."

I knew what a halo was. They're those excruciating-looking devices you may have seen somebody wearing in the mall: a ring of shiny metal that encircles the head (hence the name), supported by a cage that rests on a harness braced on the shoulders. Four large bolts run through the halo and into the patient's skull, gripping the head rigidly in place like a Christmas tree in its stand. A little crust of blood where the bolts penetrate the skin completes the picture. They look terrible, but patients tell me that after the first day or so they don't really hurt. Getting one put on, however: that hurts.

"So when does he get it?" I asked. Again, I knew the answer. It was already past noon. I was pretty sure it was Monday.

"Well," the Ortho resident replied, "it's already past noon."

"And you're in surgery."

"Yeah."

"And tomorrow?"

"Clinic. All-day clinic."

I didn't say anything. I waited a long time, biting my tongue.

"I guess we could do it tonight."

"That'd be nice."

"Unless there's an emergency, of course."

"Of course."

Of course there was. And clinic ran overtime the next day, or so I was told. Their notes on the chart (they came by each morning at five forty-five) ran to five scribbled lines, ending each time with *Plan halo. Will follow,* and a signature and pager number I couldn't quite decipher. This left me, of course, holding the bag. Not only had I one more unnecessary patient crowding my census, one more patient to see in the morning, round on, and write notes about (this during the month our team set the record for admissions to cardiology), but I also had the unpleasant responsibility of walking into Mr. Gillet's room on Tuesday and Wednesday morning to find him unhaloed, and making apologies for it.

It would have been unpleasant, at least, but for Mrs. Gillet. Her quiet grace put me in mind of faces I'd seen in old oil paintings, looking off to one side at something beyond the frame, eyes lit by what she saw there, the rest of the scene lost in dark chiaroscuro. All of which only made the situation even more intolerable, driving me to want to *do* something—and the only thing I had to offer lay in the gift of the inaccessible Ortho resident.

Wednesday I was on call again, and had pledged myself, in the brief moments between admissions, to track down the Ortho team and make them come up and put that halo on. Unfortunately, this was the day we admitted fifteen patients, as the failure clinic opened its floodgates and the Cath Lab pumped out case after case. Nobody was any too sick—the ER was blessedly free of chest pain—but the sheer volume of histories to take, physicals to perform, notes and orders to compose was overwhelming. The phone call—with its necessary sequel of waiting for the paged resident to call back—never happened.

Sometime in the late afternoon, however, I looked up from

the counter where I had been leaning, trying to absorb the salient features of yet another failure patient's complex history, and saw through the open door of Mr. Gillet's room a strange tableau: two tall men in green scrubs wielding socket wrenches around the patient's head, a tangle of chrome, and the patient's hands quivering in the air, fingers spread as if calling on the seas to part. Some time later I looked up again and the green scrubs were gone: Mr. Gillet lay propped up in his bed, his head in a halo. From the side, his nose was a hawk's beak, the rest of his face sunk in drugged sleep, but his mouth still snarled as if it remembered recent pain. I remembered him in the ER, the flash of injured pride he had been able to conjure even through the morphine. That was gone now. He looked like a strange, sad bird in a very small cage.

Still later—time on that service being marked by missed meals and sleep, I can say only that I was hungry, but not yet punchy—a nurse stopped me.

"Fourteen," she said.

She meant Mr. Gillet. "How's he doing?" I was harboring some vague hope that he was awake and asking to go home.

"He's complaining of chest pain. Ten out of ten."

"Crap," I said. The nurse looked at me. "Get an EKG."

My vague hope vanished entirely ten minutes later as I watched the red graph paper emerge from the side of the box. The squiggle on it looked better than the initial set from the ER, but that was only because the ectopy was gone. What was there instead—Mr. Gillet's souvenir of the activities of the afternoon—were T-wave inversions marching across his precordium. This is not good. T-wave inversions generally signify heart muscle that isn't getting oxygen. What I was seeing here suggested that his LAD—a major artery supplying blood to the heart's strongest muscle—was about to choke off. I looked up at the nurse. She had been reading the strip as well—upside down, as cardiology nurses can.

"You gonna move him?" she asked.

"Yeah."

"Write me some orders."

"I'll write you orders. Just get him to the Unit. Quickly," I added, with a backward glance through the door of fourteen. Gillet's beaked face lay still in its silver cage. I scratched out a set of orders and turned to the next disaster.

I DIDN'T GIVE GILLET much thought the rest of the evening, beyond seeing him settled in the CCU, and getting him scheduled as an add-on for the Cath Lab the next day. Around two in the morning the three of us—my partner Sasha, the intern Jeff, and I—were gathered at one end of the long counter, pushing stacks of paper around and trying to count up the score. We were on admission twelve for the day, we decided, but couldn't remember who was up next. I was digging in my pockets for a coin to flip when my pager went off. I swore as I tugged it from my belt, expecting to find yet again the number for the ER. I found instead the number for the CCU, followed by "911." At that moment the overhead paging system called a code in the CCU. The three of us ran.

It was perhaps thirty yards to the CCU, but by the time we got there three of the six nurses on shift were in Gillet's room, one at the head squeezing oxygen through a bag-valve mask, another compressing his chest, a third readying the crash cart. I had a moment's awareness that something was unusual—the whole thing looked too emptily staged, some kind of diorama in the Museum of Human Misery—but the scene only appeared that way for an instant and then we were in it and perspective fell apart in a surge of activity that picked us all up on its back and hurried us on.

Sasha and I had never made any formal arrangement about who did what in a code. I was the first one on the far side of the bed and started feeling the groin for a pulse. It was faint, driven solely by the nurse's compressions, but clear enough. I grabbed a finder syringe from the tray a nurse held out to me and plunged it in. Nothing. Pull back, change angle, feel for the pulse again and drive. Needle ground against bone. Again, and on this pass I saw the flash in the syringe, flung it aside and put a thumb over the welling blood while reaching for the wire. The nurse had it out already, handle turned toward me. It threaded the vein without resistance.

I had the catheter in place a minute or two later, met at each step in the process by the right item held out at the right time. No one spoke a word.

On the other side of the bed, Sasha stood with her arms folded across her chest, nodding at two nurses in turn as they pushed drugs, placed pads on the chest, and warmed up the defibrillator. Her eyes were on the monitor overhead, where green light drew lazy lines across the screen. At some point in the proceedings Anesthesia had shown up and slipped an endotracheal tube down Gillet's throat; respiratory therapy was wheeling a ventilator to the head of the bed, looping tubing through the bars of the halo and cursing at it.

"Hold compressions," Sasha said. The nurse stopped pushing on the chest. I saw for the first time that the halo was supported by a broad sheet of plastic backed with sheepskin that covered the upper half of the chest: the nurse had to get her hands underneath it to press; with each compression Gillet's head bobbed up and down, up and down. He was out, his eyes blank at the ceiling. The nurse at my elbow was hooking up the ports of my catheter, pushing one of the blunt syringes of epinephrine. We were all staring at the monitor above the bed, the long horizontal drift of asystole. As the second amp of atropine ran in, the lines all leapt to life, frantic peaks filling the screen.

"V-fib," a nurse said quietly.

"Paddles," Sasha replied in the same voice, taking the offered handgrips of the defibrillator from the nurse as she spoke.

"Clear," she said quietly, and thumbed the button.

David Gillet's body rose from the mattress, hung for a moment, collapsed. On the screen we saw scrambled green light settle for a moment, a rhythm emerge. Then the peaked lines consolidated into a high picket fence.

"V-tach," said the nurse, and turned up the power on the defibrillator.

"Clear," said Sasha. The body arched and fell again.

It went on for twelve more minutes (we knew this later, as we reviewed the printed strips of telemetry paper, trying to reconstruct what had gone on), Gillet's heart flying through one arrhythmia after another. Each time we responded it would settle briefly into sinus rhythm before flinging out again into some lethal variation, until finally, after two grams of magnesium sulfate and another round of shocks, it found a rhythm and held it through another flurry of activity when his systolics dropped to the sixties, then rallied on a minimal infusion of dopamine. And through all of this, as the atmosphere in the room maintained its eerie calm, the nurses kept up their surreal economy of gesture, and Sasha intoned the ritual of the ACLS algorithm, I felt my own adrenaline surging through the night's fatigue in an approach to exultation. It was almost beautiful.

This, I thought as we left the room, the lines on the monitor dancing their steady dance, the ventilator measuring breath and time to its own slower rhythm, this is what a code should be. A clean thing. A beautiful thing. The patient hadn't died.

THE REST OF THE NIGHT was anticlimax, of course. There was a note to write (there is always a note to write), for which we had to puzzle some time over the strips churned out by the telemetry system, the notes scribbled on a paper towel recording what drugs had been given when, the values called over the phone from Core Lab and written in black marker on the leg of a nurse's scrubs. There was the call to the wife: I had to temper my enthusiasm as I searched for words to use when calling from the CCU at 2:35 in the morning. She took the news well enough, asked if I thought she needed to come now. I assured her he was stable. I assured her everything was under control; I had anticipated the code, I realized, when I moved him to the CCU. He was in the safest possible place. "In the morning, then," she said softly.

"In the morning," I agreed, and turned to the call room at last, where I spent perhaps forty-five minutes on my back, replaying the code against the springs of the empty bunk above me, until my pager went off again and this time it was the ER. And then around five another code on 4 West, where we found a man bleeding from a ruptured arterial graft and I had to threaten him with death if he did not hold still while I put yet another catheter in yet another groin, and this time there were fourteen nurses in the room, all shouting at once, so that I had to bellow over them to be heard as I requested, repeatedly, the proper catheter kit, something big enough to pour in fluid as fast as he was losing it. The patient was alive when I saw him last, a scared and tousled surgery intern kneeling right on top of him to hold pressure as the entire ungainly assemblage—patient, intern, and tree of IV bags— wheeled out the door to the OR. Back to normal life, I said to Sasha as we trudged back to the cardiology ward. Whether she knew what I was talking about I couldn't say, and didn't really care. I was still warmed by a vague sense of something right having happened. Mr. Gillet had coded, coded beautifully, and he had survived. We had done everything right.

THE NEXT MORNING ON ROUNDS, we were congratulated for our management of Mr. Gillet's arrest, although there was an ominous pH value from a blood gas obtained early on in the event that occasioned some shaking of heads. He had not responded since the code, being content to lie there unconscious in his halo, his chest rising and falling in response to the ventilator's efforts. But his vital signs were stable, his labs from the four a.m. draw were looking good, and I had my hopes. No longer for an early discharge, but I was hopeful, all the same.

I shared these hopes with Mrs. Gillet when she arrived at seven. She stood at the bedside looking down, and her eyes were wet, her mouth unstably mobile. She reached out almost to touch the bars supporting the halo, down one of the threaded rods that pierced her husband's skin above the temple, almost touched there, then withdrew. "Is this the . . . thing? What do they call it?"

I was silent a moment.

"A halo," I said finally. "They call it a halo."

"Ah," she said.

I left her at the bedside, Mrs. Gillet with one hand through the chrome that cradled her husband's head.

DAVID GILLET DIED FIVE days later, having never regained consciousness. As each day passed and he gave no sign of mental activity, eventually it became clear that not all of him had survived the code. Mrs. Gillet decided, once pneumonia set in, to withdraw support. I had to agree. Even though I had anticipated the pneumonia, and was pretty sure I could get him through it, I had to agree it was for the best. Much as I wanted to keep him around.

He had become something unreal for me—something

beautiful, like a work of art, but unreal. Amid all the mess and squalor of the hospital, with its blind random unraveling of lives, in their patient dignity and kindness he and his wife stood apart. In his case, for a little while at least, everything had gone exactly as it should have. The perfect code. And it hadn't made any difference. No difference at all. I pulled his tube early in the afternoon, after a bedside service, and took my place at the wall while the usual drama worked to its conclusion.

She sent me a card that Christmas, Mrs. Gillet. I kept it for a while, until it vanished in the clutter on my desk. She had written a text inside, something from the New Testament I had admired at the bedside service, but soon forgot. I do remember vividly the picture on the card. It was like her: sober, attractive. It showed a medieval nativity scene, all saints and angels with their burnished golden ovals overhead. Their faces were sorrowful in profile, as if anticipating what will crown that rosy newborn, perfection laid in straw, with pain in time to come.

WHEN
I
WAS
WRONG

I WAS STILL IN THE PARKING GARAGE WHEN MY pager went off. The callback number was the ER. Naturally I was annoyed. This was week three of my first ICU rotation as a resident, and I was cranky with stress and lack of sleep, but even without that there was reason to be annoyed. The MAO is supposed to stall admissions between six and seven in the morning, out of courtesy to the team coming on call, which is busy getting ready to round. But the problem with critical care medicine is that some things can't wait down in the ER while the rhythms of hospital life play out. So, annoyed but not surprised, I returned the page.

THE MAO, WHO HAD been up all night, was inexcusably cheery. "You're gonna love this one," he said.

"What?" I said flatly.

"Be that way. But you're still gonna thank me."

I grunted, having lost a parking space to an incoming medical student.

"Anyway, what we got here is a sixty-two-year-old lady with a big ICH, she's—"

"Neurosurgery go home already?" I knew the futility of the question, but I had to make the attempt.

"Neurosurgery's seen her and signed off. They said . . ." I heard paper shuffle. "Here: 'prognosis is dismal.' They used the *d*-word. It's a chip shot."

I grunted noncommittally. I didn't want to involve myself in the MAO's creepy good cheer any more than I had to.

"She stable?"

"For now. Vented, obtunded, holding her pressures."

"Family?"

"Family's all here, I've talked to them, they seem reasonable, but I left the dirty work for you. You do it so well."

I ignored him, grunting one more time as I finally wedged my car into a space vacated by a departing night nurse. "Don't let the family get away."

"Don't worry. From the look of things, they're here for the duration."

IT WAS ALMOST TEN before I made my way toward the ER. In the meantime, in a none-too-surprising violation of custom, the ER had decided to send her up to the ICU before I'd had a chance to see her, so as the elevator opened I found myself facing a gurney bearing a large, unconscious form, a ventilator, a nurse, and a respiratory therapist. My doorway survey told me this patient wasn't going to be on my service very long. I heard the echo of the MAO's breezy chuckle and suppressed a grimace.

"This the lady with the head bleed?"

"You got it," the nurse said, leaning hard to get the gurney into motion. It lurched out of the elevator, dragging the vent and IV pole behind it. I lent a hand, swiveling the assemblage out into the corridor.

"The family coming up?"

"They're probably in your waiting room already."

We got the patient into a room, settled a few questions about the vent, and I spent a minute rummaging through her chart, jotting down a name, age, and record number. There was a brown jacket with a CT from an outside hospital. I held it up to the fluorescents overhead. You didn't need to be a neuroradiologist to call this one: there was an inky cloud larger than a golf ball low down on the right side of her brain. It was blood. It also marked a region of dead and dying brain cells, killed by pressure from the expanding mass. With a bleed like this, there's essentially nothing to be done. There's no avenue of approach for the surgeons that won't destroy more than they could save. If the bleeding doesn't stop, eventually the rising pressure in the skull will extrude the brain through a narrow opening in the membrane that supports the cerebrum within the skull. This process is called herniating: it's inexorably fatal, but not all that common. From the looks of this one, she didn't seem about to herniate. But it didn't look like she was going to survive, either: the hole in her brain was big, and it was low, down where the essential circuitry of life is wired.

———

I WAS MARSHALING ALL of this largely automatically, as I moved from the smoky shadows of the CT to the patient herself, flashing light in her eyes, tapping on her joints, trying to elicit signs of withdrawal from pain. I wiggled the ventilator tube and she grimaced, slightly: the right side of her mouth curled back in a vague snarl. But the left side was motionless, slack, a slice of eye visible below the lid. With a last glance at the monitor, where a green light kept tracing a steady heartbeat, I made my way out to the waiting room.

AT THAT HOUR OF the day, the waiting room is usually empty, the TV set muttering to itself in a waste of polished blond wood and dusty fabric plants. This morning almost every chair was full. There were children sitting listlessly on the floor. Teenagers slumped in uncomfortable postures, small knots of couples and siblings and cousins and aunts and neighbors and friends and one frail-looking old man wearing a baseball cap with the name of a feed supplier on its stained green front.

"Are you the Wallace family?" I knew the answer, of course, but the sheer size of the crowd had me taken aback. I had a sense of things possibly escaping my control.

From the assembled multitude there came a rumble of assent.

I moved into the room, not sure where to position myself. "I'm one of the doctors taking care of Mrs. Wallace now," I began. I looked at the frail old man. "Are you Mr. . . . ?"

He looked at me with an expression of absolute incomprehension, his head wavering on his skinny neck. "That's him," somebody said. "That's her husband."

I moved closer to him, propping myself on the edge of an end table. "Mr. Wallace?"

He nodded.

I identified myself again, and then paused. I did that partly to give myself a moment to think, partly to let them know that something bad was coming.

"I'm terribly sorry to have to tell you this," I began. A low murmur ran around the room. "I've just come from the intensive care unit, and though I'm just beginning my assessment, I'm afraid that I have to agree with the specialists who saw her in the emergency room."

At some point in my training, I was told that it was useful in situations such as this to say "specialists." It lends authority. It helps people take in the facts they don't want to know.

"From the tests they've done, and my own exam, I'm afraid her outlook at this point is very bad."

I stopped again to let it sink in.

"I can't say at this point if she's going to live."

Another murmur. "That's in God's hands," a voice said, followed by, "That's right. That's right," from all around the room.

"That's right," I agreed. I have little knowledge of God, but in situations like this I've found it's useful to agree. "Her fate is out of our hands."

Another long silence.

"Or I wish it was, anyway." This elicited another murmur,

audibly puzzled. The old man was looking at me as though I were a hallucination.

I sighed, a completely unscripted sigh.

"The problem is," I went on, "we're keeping her alive. We have a machine breathing for her." I looked around the room. There must have been at least thirty of them, all looking at me. "And tubes running in and out of her. She's on life support. She can't speak for herself now. She needs you to speak for her." Another murmur of assent. "And the question she's going to need you to start thinking about—and may need you to answer very soon—is this: Do you think she would have wanted all this?"

A prolonged rumble. The old man in front of me gave no sign he'd heard a word. His eyes—a startling, cloudy blue—weren't tracking on anything. The tremor of his head went on as though hidden devices were gently stirring him. The rumble rose around us to a scattering of broken words, until finally, from close at hand, a stout woman in her forties said, "What'd happen if you turn off the machine?"

"Then it would truly be in God's hands." As soon as the words were out of my mouth, I wanted to call them back. I have no business invoking God.

But my words called forth another murmur of assent. "Turn it off," a voice in the back of the room said. There was another rumble. "She didn't want all this."

This was, of course, what any resident in the ICU would want to hear, and I was relieved to hear it, if a little surprised to hear it so soon. To some extent, this relief is only a humane response to an inhuman situation. In too many cases we keep

bodies alive in a way that is only cruel, cruel in direct proportion not only to its futility, but also to the manifold distresses,
large and small, physical and spiritual, inflicted by technologies
that only put off the inevitable end. To another extent, always
there, undeniable but uncomfortable all the same, this relief is
a response to the inhuman load of work and worry that comes
with the ICU, caring for too many patients and making too
many decisions, and too often failing in our task.

But this was too fast. The atmosphere in the room was a
little too much like a revival meeting. The enthusiasm was
making me nervous. I stood, and started to back toward the
door. "You all need time to discuss this. I'll be here if you have
questions. I just want you to remember that the decision has
to be yours. We can't decide, and she can't tell us. So you have
to speak for her."

I scuttled out of the room as fast as I could.

I DON'T KNOW HOW many times I've given that speech, or
some version of it, in one small room or another, in one hospital or another. It's a speech that needs speaking, God knows.
No one gets up in the morning expecting to end the day in
the ICU, but every day those beds get filled. And very few of
the people in them can tell me how they feel about what we're
doing to them.

I know how I feel about it. During morning rounds one
day late in my intern year, after a night in which all fourteen
patients under my care had seemed to be doing their level best
to die, I came out of the haze to hear another exhausted intern

make a suggestion regarding a patient whose acute pancreatitis had caused her lungs to fill with fluid. The doctor in charge, to whom the suggestion was addressed, had thought for a moment, then replied judiciously, "We could do that. It *might* kill her." In my delicate state of mind, I missed the irony of that remark. What my overwrought imagination heard instead was a conversation coming from an ICU in some horrible parallel universe, where the goal was not to save the patient, but to kill her, as slowly as possible. Looking around the unit, at the glassed cubicles where bodies hung from a network of tubing and wires strung over the abyss, it occurred to me that, if such had been our aim, the place would not look all that different. It would not look different at all.

But after rotating through the unit several times, I came to understand what my peers were saying when they said they enjoy the ICU, even though I knew I would never share the feeling. There is a simplicity about unit work, a freedom from the messy problems of discharge and placement, even from many of the refinements of therapy. The things we do to people there are for the most part brutal, simple, and effective. We sustain breath with an adjustable air pump. We support blood pressure with any combination of four different drugs. We fight off infection by the simple means of hosing down the patient with the three or four antibiotics necessary to cover the entire spectrum of known pathogens. The patient doesn't talk back. The patient doesn't move. The nurses are generally brilliant. As medicine, it's relatively simple. And there is a pure and uncomplicated pleasure in taking a patient who is minutes away from death and dragging him out of darkness into light.

The problem, of course, is that sometimes you fall short of that goal. Too often, we're able to rescue somebody from death, but can't quite bring him back to life. People get stuck in that horrible twilight in between. And while they may not be able to tell you, it's difficult to escape the impression that, even if they could, they wouldn't want to thank you. This is something that can be difficult for people to understand, especially when the patient is someone who just that morning, or the week before, had been a fully living, fully functional, and deeply loved human being.

We practice a scrupulous ethics in my hospital. Patients decide the limits of their care. If they can't talk, the family tells us what to do. And no matter what I think of their decision, I am bound to respect their wishes, up to the point where my efforts are clearly futile, and then the question is moot: at that point, usually, the patient speaks in the only way left to him, by dying despite everything I can do. Whenever the decision is taken out of my hands, I feel relieved. Who would want the power to decide?

AROUND THE MIDDLE OF the afternoon, I was down in the ED working up a new admission (eighty-three-years-old, living alone, found unconscious on the floor with a core temperature of 107 degrees, and now barely holding her pressures on ten micrograms of dopamine) when I was paged to the ICU. The Wallace family wanted to speak to me. In the interim, Muriel Wallace's condition hadn't changed in any significant way. There was no sign her stroke had progressed. Her blood pressure was stable, her heartbeat solid as a rock; as I prepared to meet the family, this, and the way she was breathing over the vent, made me slightly uneasy—the way one always is in the hospital when things don't progress according to plan.

"Breathing over the vent," means the patient is taking breaths without the aid of the ventilator. Ventilator management can be complicated; in patients whose lungs are severely damaged, the subtleties of their settings become a matter of art as much as science. But for most patients, as for Mrs. Wallace, the machine was there simply because she was intubated, and it's hard to breathe through a narrow tube without mechanical aid. The tube itself was there only because she was unconscious: she was intubated for airway protection, and the vent was on minimal support only, supplying breaths twelve times a minute, and giving a helpful push on any breath the patient started drawing on her own. Even on her own breaths, she was drawing in more than the vent supplied. Odds were good that if I were to extubate her, she would go on breathing.

This made me uneasy, I say, as I found the family and ushered them into the conference room across the hall—dozens of them squeezing in until the room was walled with standing, silent figures. Around the table by some tacit agreement most of the elders had arranged themselves in some order of precedence. Mr. Wallace sat at the far end, wobbling, unseeing, fragile. I didn't have the time to figure out for myself just where this plot seemed to be headed. With her massive bleed yoked to her unimpaired respiratory drive, Muriel Wallace was entering a gray area.

But I was running on autopilot, feeling pressure to move

on to some next step in the process. My pager had buzzed twice while the family was filing in. One of the new admissions was crashing. I had a sense of events piling up just outside the room.

A large, stout woman to Mr. Wallace's right—unmistakably Muriel's daughter—spoke.

"We've been discussing," she began. "Like you said."

I nodded encouragingly. She went on. "We'd like to begin by saying how much we appreciate . . ." She paused here, and the silence filled itself with muttered assents. "Appreciate," she said again, "all the care you've shown our mother."

"And aunt."

"And sister."

"Amen."

"We truly do," the woman went on. I could hear a "but" looming, and settled myself, trying to remember that I wasn't here to argue. I wasn't pushing an agenda. I was here to help. My pager was going off again.

"But." And her gaze swept around the room. No one stirred. "We have some questions."

I murmured some polite invitation.

"What," the woman began, "are our options here?"

I thought for a minute. "I suppose there are three." But that wasn't right. I was skipping something. "But before we discuss them, I thought you'd want to know how she's doing."

Yes, they sighed.

"She's unchanged."

The sigh flowed out of the room.

"She's not better and she's not worse." This seemed to me

to sum up the salient features of the case. I plowed on with details.

"She's still unconscious. I have no idea when or if she'll wake up." I paused, letting the room absorb the sound of my voice. "Meanwhile, she's still on the breathing machine." I stopped, wondering where to go next. "But she's not using it." This elicited some stirring, eyebrows rising, nods exchanging, heads shaking. "She's breathing in and out without any help from the machine."

"What does that mean?"

It was messy was what it meant. But I wasn't sure how to say that. "It means, basically, that her stroke hasn't gotten any worse. The reflexes in the base of her brain, the parts that control breathing, they haven't been hit. We could take her off the machine right now and she'd probably do fine." No, that wasn't right. "Fine" wasn't right at all. But the words were out.

"Then let's do it," a voice said. The daughter stabbed him with a look, and turned to me.

"Is that one of our options?"

"Yes. It is. But there's a problem. With what's happened to her, it's very likely that she can't control the muscles in her throat anymore. All the reflexes that we use to keep from choking, to keep things from going down the wrong way—those don't work anymore. We'll need to do some more tests, but it's very likely that if we take the tube out, eventually she'll choke, inhale something she shouldn't, and get pneumonia."

More solemn nods from around the table; glances shifting side to side. I went on. "If that's the case, then our options would be: to keep her the way she is now, to pull the tube out, and"— for a moment I considered referring to God again, but thought better of it—"let nature take its course. Or, if tests show us she needs it, we could have the surgeons put a permanent breathing tube in here." I gestured to my own throat just above the sternal notch. "It's called a tracheostomy, and it would allow her to breathe on her own. It would also offer some protection against choking."

I stopped, not so much letting things sink in as wondering myself where we were going. I was thinking of how long it would take all this to unfold: days and days. And to what end?

"This breathing tube," the daughter asked, "is that a big operation? Will she stand up to it?"

"She shouldn't have any trouble."

Another woman, another daughter from the looks of her, chipped in from down the table. "And can she go home after that?"

That was another question. I paused a minute, this time judging the effect—going for an effect, I realized. What was I trying to do here? "I don't know," I said. "There's no way of knowing for sure. But I doubt it. From what we've seen so far, the damage is so severe, it's unlikely she'll ever rise from that bed again. Usually, with this kind of injury, you're looking at a life in a nursing home—"

Mutterings of protest. Under the glare of the daughter, they died away.

"A nursing home would really be the only place that could care for her. Dealing with somebody so severely paralyzed is hard work. There's constant care involved."

"We can do that," somebody said.

Don't argue, I told myself. "It's very hard," was all I said. "But that's not the issue we need to resolve. Not right now. The question you all need to decide is, would she want that? If all we can buy her is a little time—with frequent infections, bed sores, being unable to do anything for herself—do you think that's what she would want?"

As I said this, I could feel myself becoming increasingly uncomfortable. Not with the question itself: it's a common enough question, and one that needs to be asked—sometimes. As I listened to the sound of my voice dying away in the room, even the echoes struck me as wrong. Wrong and wrong and wrong: mistakes seemed to be showering out of me like sparks from a Catherine wheel. Listen to me, I thought: It sounds like I'm pleading with them to let her die. Like I *want* this woman to die.

Well, of course, on some level I wanted something close. There was nothing complicated or remarkable about that. Any resident who is remotely honest will tell you we become, if not comfortable, at least familiar with the sensation of wanting patients to die. We feel that way because they're going to die anyway, usually, and we know that, out of the available options, dying quickly is the best that could happen to them. But it's also better for us. There's the rub. It saves them agony, but it seems to save us something as well: the exhaustion of watching, of causing nothing but pain as we struggle to forestall the inevitable.

Of course, it doesn't really save us even that. Whatever hospitals once were, they are now largely places where people come to die. If they're not at death's door we rush them back home;

only the dying linger, but in this parallel universe every dying patient is quickly replaced by another. The house staff come to see the ICU as the place where we manage that exchange, again and again and again. The feeling is understandable. It's also, thank God, temporary, fading like bad dreams with the light of day as we get more sleep, more time with our patients, as we move up the hierarchy so that we're not the ones actively, physically, holding off death just a few seconds more.

So there I was, using all the rhetorical tricks I had at my command, I feared, to seem to push this family into pulling the plug on my patient. Was I really doing that? It would be better for the patient, after all.

And it was my job, I told myself, to help them face up to a reality most of us would rather deny. Too few of us arrive at the hospital with a duly signed and witnessed DNR order in our hands. Too few of us have the conversation with our families. And nobody out there seems to understand that the survival we have to offer is sometimes worse than—I had been going to say "death," but I don't know enough about death to use it in a comparison. Worse than what? Worse than I want to give? Perhaps it's that. I would save everyone if I could, but it's a sorry gift I have to offer, sometimes. Life in a puddle of urine, bones laid bare as the immobile flesh turns black and rots away, long hours passing while a call for something simple—a drink of water, a runny nose wiped clean—goes unanswered. I didn't want that life for Muriel Wallace, for any of my patients, for anybody.

But with every unassisted breath Muriel Wallace took, I was beginning to understand that what I wanted did not matter. My rhetoric did not matter, except insofar as it might impose my half-baked wishes on events. Muriel Wallace's life was following its own plot. It had always been that way, I knew, but just then the reality of it left me feeling bleak, uncertain of where to go next. And the entire family was still looking at me.

There were more questions, which I did my best to answer, talking on autopilot about infections, fiber endoscopies, and skilled nursing. While the family threshed through the matter, discussing things I had no business hearing, I excused myself. They would let me know. I went across the hall and back into the Unit, moving through the noise of the nursing station to the dark and relatively quiet room where Muriel Wallace lay. She was still: a big, still woman with white plastic tubes taped to her face. Gently, I jostled the end of the endotracheal tube. No response. Out of habit more than any actual curiosity, I put my stethoscope to her chest: air moving in and out, backed by the rhythmic thud of the living. Her left arm was limp, utterly flaccid, falling when I let it go in a straight drop to the bed. A big, still woman lying motionless in bed.

ANY PATIENT IN A HOSPITAL, when we take their clothes away and lay them in a bed, starts to lose identity; after a few days, they all start to merge into a single passive body, distinguishable (if even then) only by the illnesses that brought them there. In the ICU, with consciousness gone as well, there is rarely a trace of personality left behind. Spirit itself comes from a machine. The body remains behind, but all too often it's a husk, doing the work of living for nobody's benefit. It's impossible to know what's going on in there. It's impossible to read how the body came to be there, what life it left behind. Just the rise and fall of the chest, the slow accumulation of data as labs and vital signs and consults and imaging fill up the chart, telling nothing about the person they surround.

But the question of Muriel Wallace and her care had become a question not of medicine but of an unknowable will. What would Muriel want? It was clear enough that she had had a stroke that should have killed her, and was certainly, I thought, going to leave her hemiplegic forever. She had to look forward to a future of infections of the lung, of the bladder, and then the slow ripening of sores. There was no easy solution for the problem of being Muriel. None that I could give.

And none that she could give, either. We go along in our lives, making plans, expecting things will continue the way they have, confident that we know what we want, what we might and might not have. But lives don't go like that: no matter what we will for ourselves or others, time hides abrupt and wrenching dislocations, moments that change everything. Muriel had been through one of those moments. And after that, what anybody knew, what anybody wanted, was irrelevant. More and more the facts seemed to tell us that she was going to live. She was going to have to live with what happened to her. I picked her limp arm back up, folded it across her, covered it with the thin hospital sheet. She gave no sign. The ventilator heaved a sigh as I left the room.

I WISH I COULD provide something neater to end this piece. It didn't end neatly—hasn't, for all I know, ended at all. Muriel survived our care. She did develop pneumonia, but anyone will in her situation: we were waiting for it, and she responded within a day or two to antibiotics. Later, she woke up, just as her family had hoped. She even greeted me one morning with a half-wide half grimace, a strong grip with her good right hand. She nodded vigorously to almost any suggestion, nodded and squeezed about getting the trach and the G-tube, and as soon as her fever was down, on two successive days she got them both installed, and we were able to wean her off the vent without a problem, and the nurses started to teach her family how to pour into her G-tube the cans of gray-green liquid that from now on would be her food. Then, her need for intensive monitoring past, we transferred her to one of the general medicine services, who would manage her care until she had a bed somewhere beyond our walls.

AS LUCK WOULD HAVE IT, I followed her a day or so later, rotating off the ICU to general medicine. My first day on the service, the family greeted me like lost kin. They were no longer a collective tableau of grief, resolving instead into individuals, who spoke, gestured, laughed. That day they were laughing—gently, happily—at me. Pulling me into the room during rounds, they interrupted the intern's presentation with a delighted—and slightly ironic—demonstration of Muriel's ability to move the toes of her left foot, the ghost of a grip she had developed in her left hand. Muriel beamed at me as she showed us what she could do. The intern beamed and completed her presentation. The plan for Muriel, for the remainder of her stay, was physical therapy, speech therapy, occupational therapy, and social work consultation for placement. The family had agreed to place her in a nursing home for rehab, confident that it would be a short sojourn before returning to the life she had known. I beamed back at them, nodding blindly, not looking at the figure still splayed so limply on the bed.

ON THE DAY OF her transfer to the nursing facility, Muriel was found unresponsive, and hypotensive to the eighties over forties. It seemed for a moment that her story had taken another turn, or turned back, anyway, into the usual course of things in the hospital. She spent that night in the ICU again, getting a liter of fluid. That fluid may or may not have been responsible for the recovery of her pressures. At any rate, something turned this climax into peripeteia: the story continued, again taking its own path to its own end. For now, at least, she rebounded. What set her back in the first place? Nobody knew. Things like this were to be expected. By the next day she was back on the general medicine service, and the day after that, her family took her away. I didn't see her go.

In the years since then, I've thought about her often, wondering how she's getting along. It would be easy enough to find out how her story finally ended, but I've resisted. I'd like to leave her the way she is, lying in that bed with her family so pleased, beaming at me because I was wrong.

HEART
FAILURE

*Let the lamp affix
its beam*

MARIE P WAS ADMITTED TO THE CARDIOLOGY service from the Failure Clinic one day in February, a three-hundred-pound woman with a history of non-ischemic cardiomyopathy. Her heart was failing. I was a resident, one of nine staffing the CCU that month, just past the halfway point of my residency. It was my second rotation through the CCU that year.

The CCU—cardiac care unit—was a critical care service, in which teams of residents rotated call not every fourth night, as the practice was on other services, but every third. This turned an otherwise grueling month—all months in the hospital are grueling—into a marathon. On the day Marie came in from the Failure Clinic, I was two weeks into the rotation and was already exhausted. Or maybe something more. After two years of constant call, I was empty.

It was our bad luck to be admitting on the day of Failure Clinic.

"Heart failure" is a fairly common diagnosis. It sounds ominous, and it is, but the reality is less dramatic than the words suggest. It does not mean, for instance, that the heart is about to stop. The disease is actually more of a chronic condition, what used to be called the dropsy, in which the heart, weakened by a poor blood supply or alcohol or untreated hypertension—the list is long—can no longer drive blood around the body as well as it should. Fluid backs up, one place or another. If the weakness is primarily on the heart's left side, fluid accumulates in the lungs: you cough, get short of breath, can't lie down flat without a sensation of smothering. If it's on the right side, your legs and belly swell, the liver stretches; the veins on your neck stand out, pulsing. And because the whole circulation is connected, failure on one side eventually becomes failure on both. At that point the patient enters the terminal phase. Then "failure" comes to mean what we usually mean by it, like "breakdown" or "collapse." But this can take years.

The culprit in this persistent flooding is not the heart so much as the foolish kidney, which continues to do its job of regulating the body's fluid levels, but does so in an increasingly misleading milieu. As the heart's output drops off, the kidney senses decreased flow and in response holds on to water as tightly as it can: your weight climbs, your ankles swell, you start to feel congested: you're suffering an exacerbation of congestive heart failure. When your doctor gets a look at those puffy ankles and hears the crackles in the lungs, she calls up the cardiology service and sends over what the admitting resident will describe to the intern as "another damn tune-up." Marie was in for a tune-up, a four- to five-day process in which we wring out all that extra fluid, undoubtedly the dullest medical intervention a hospital can provide. Marie had gone through this so many times before that it was all I could do to lift her chart—heavy in proportion to her obesity, packed with details of prior tune-ups, diagnostic studies, lab values, and a pervading sense of futility . . . which was increasingly how my own fatigue had come to feel.

By the time I met her, Marie P had long since passed the point where the occasional tune-up would suffice; she had been discharged from her last admission on a permanent infusion of dobutamine, without which her heart would simply grind to a halt. She got it through a Permaport installed over her collarbone, and a pump that followed her everywhere.

What we were supposed to do with her was simply crank up the settings on the pump and see how much fluid we could draw off. And although this was not without risk (side effects of dobutamine include lethal arrhythmias), this is not the stuff of which careers in cardiology are made. My partner on the service that month, Alex, was applying for fellowships in cardiology. I took Marie under my care.

Such as it was. She arrived on the floor sometime in the late afternoon, competing for my attention with a man having a genuine heart attack and a woman whose aorta seemed to be disintegrating. When the nurse informed me of her arrival, I scratched out a set of generic orders and returned to the gray, sweating fellow who was heading for the cath lab. I didn't lay eyes on Marie until after ten that night. Her room was dark, her vital signs were stable. I should have awakened her and repeated the intern's history and physical exam. But as I listened to her snoring, propped up in her bed so that her lungs wouldn't fill from her internal seeps and springs, I thought about the two dozen prior admissions documented in her chart, and how little changed from one to the next. I didn't wake her up.

FOR THE NEXT SEVERAL DAYS, Marie hovered vaguely on the margins of my attention. She was a tune-up, someone whose progress I would measure in liters of urine. She was a body to examine each morning, a set of labs and vitals to record, a very simple story to present each day on rounds. She herself remained tucked into the end room on the intermediate care unit, a fat little woman with a tremulous manner and a wedge of tight pallid curls that made her head, from sharp chin to spreading jowls to the bed-flattened top of her curls, a cone. I hated her.

"Hated" may be too strong a word. At that time, I hadn't the energy for hatred. Certainly I didn't like her. I think it was primarily the way she whimpered when I examined her. The sound she made grated on me, partly because I didn't believe I was hurting her, also because that was all she would do— pucker her face around a sharp gasp, never looking at me or blaming me. After a week of this, my physical exam dwindled to a cursory prod at her ankles and the briefest auscultation of her chest.

There was also the issue of her Xanax. Xanax, alprazolam, is a tranquilizer, a member of the family of benzodiazepines, the most familiar member of which is Valium. It is probably the most addictive drug in its class, primarily because of the speed with which it enters and exits the system. Users get a buzz off it, and four hours later they withdraw. Unsurprisingly, Marie was a Xanax addict. People with syndromes that cause shortness of breath tend to be anxious—we're wired that way—and often wind up on benzos. Emotionally, at least, the drug becomes as important to them as oxygen. And although none of us balks at supplying oxygen to a patient feeling short of breath—even if we suspect the sensation to be imaginary—there is something about the Xanax addict that can inspire contempt. It did in me at that time in my life.

So she was obese, she whimpered, and she had a drug habit. She also had a heart that beat with perhaps a fifth of the strength it should have. Had she been a younger woman, she would have been listed for transplant. But at her age, with her obesity and other problems, she was in a holding mode, circling the drain in rings that seemed still, at this point, so wide that the central vortex was only a dimple on the horizon. This pass through the hospital was just another one of those slow circles, routine, intolerably so. Had I known this was to be her last admission, I might have regarded her differently.

It was on day five that the dullness of things broke. That day, rounds took longer than they should have, and I was due in clinic by one. By the time we reached Marie's door, I was so tired of standing I had forgotten most of what I had known about her. I searched my notes through a fog of fatigue. All that emerged was data: her weight so many kilograms, her urine output so many mLs. I looked up to find the attending frowning.

Not at me, thank god.

"What do you think is going on here?" she asked me.

I thought furiously. "Nothing," I said, glancing back at my notes. Over the past few days, despite heroic doses of furosemide, we hadn't wrung more than a liter of fluid from her overloaded circulation. "That's a problem, isn't it?"

"Yes," she said. "What's standard of care here?"

"Metolazone," I said, naming a diuretic often used to increase the effect of furosemide. "And crank the dobutamine."

I had answered correctly, because she nodded, still thinking. "What's tele show?"

She was asking about the continuous telemetry of the patient's EKG. "Nothing significant."

"Okay," she said, jerking her thumb upward. "Get cranking. She's losing ground here."

And so we moved on to the next patient, and by one p.m. I had signed out to the on-call intern that Marie was to be a liter negative by morning, and if not to hit her with an extra 120 IV at four a.m., but to watch her K.

The next morning we were on call again. I spent the half hour before rounds checking up on the three patients I was carrying going into call. I left Marie to last, my reluctance to enter her room being by this time nearly insuperable. In response to my usual question, she gave her usual answer. "Terrible. I feel so weak, Doctor. Just so weak and shaky." She said this in her usual tremulous voice, waving the back of her hand over her face to express her weakness. I couldn't help but notice, uncharitably, her breakfast tray, every bowl and plate stripped clean to the last sheen of grease. Her vital signs were stable, and her urine output had indeed picked up: not the entire liter we had hoped for, but most of it. It was with a feeling of hope—I might discharge her soon—that I left her room for a last check of labs before rounds.

But what I saw in the labs wasn't good. Overnight, Marie's serum creatinine—the general indicator of the kidney's ability to clear wastes—had almost doubled. Worse, her potassium—the "K" I had asked the intern to watch—was over six. The number was highlighted on the screen in red. We watch potassium generally in hospitalized patients: it's a critical element, its level easily perturbed, and too wide a deviation can throw the heart's rhythm awry. A patient on dobutamine with a potassium greater than six was not something I wanted to present on rounds. I had three minutes to find a nurse and order the four different things that would take care of this. As I was scribbling the orders on the chart, somewhere in the back of my head I was processing the other half of this story, the one I could do nothing about. Her heart was overloaded with fluid her kidneys could no longer expel. And now, under the burden of her failing heart, her kidneys were beginning to fail as well.

I was a minute late for the start of rounds.

As another long day of call ground into motion, I carried with me through the morning's rituals a bleak sensation of change about to happen. Or perhaps, with the shift of a few numbers on a computer display, it already had, crossing over from the well-worn track Marie's history had followed so faithfully for so long, to the other routine that plots the hospital's daily round, the inexorable slippage into death. Marie's electrolyte abnormality was significant not because it put her at risk of sudden death (although it did). The real significance was that the routine tune-up was over. Our only means of lightening the load on Marie's heart had failed. This much, at least, had become brutally clear by rounds the next morning, even after another sleepless night.

When we reached her doorway I presented the data, and ground to a halt. I had no idea what came next.

The attending turned to the fellow.

"Now what?"

The fellow tugged at his lower lip. "I think we need to Swann her."

The attending nodded. The fellow turned to me and said, "Move her to the Unit. We'll Swann her after rounds."

My legs sagged. I'd been up all night—all month, it seemed—and it was now ten forty-five; we'd been rounding since eight, and still had seven patients to see. It would be a miracle if we finished by noon. I wanted to go home, of course. I wanted to sleep, to stop thinking, more than anything else to stop thinking about Marie P. Beyond that, I hated the Swann. I hated the Swann because it takes at least an hour to set up, and hours more to thread a catheter into the jugular, through the heart, and into the lung. And then the fellow wants to spend hours more taking readings, before finally some decision emerges from the procedure, one I would be responsible for acting upon. I didn't want to hang around to run scut afterward. Marie was just supposed to be a tune-up. She wasn't supposed to take this much time.

It fell to me, as the resident, to float the Swann. Sometime around one p.m., the hour when, after a night on my feet, my higher functions start to wink out like so many overused lamps, I stood at the head of Marie's new bed in the CCU, hieratically gowned and masked. Marie herself had disappeared under a wad of sterile green towels (it had required four milligrams of Ativan to get her to hold still for this), from which her tiny, rhythmic snores could be heard.

As I approached her neck with a four-inch needle, the landmarks by which I was supposed to find the internal jugular vein were awash in flesh, but I was lucky, and on the first pass an abrupt flash of blood swirled into the barrel of the syringe in deep purple arabesques. "Got it," I announced. The fellow, whose customary moroseness had taken on an overlay of anxiety, rattled out unnecessary advice. "Hold your finger over the hub, that's it, don't lose it, now advance the wire, good," rising in volume and frequency as the nurse on my right fed me a long, skinny tube, which I advanced into Marie's neck. This went on for some time, until the fellow barked, "Stop. We got a wedge."

"That's a wedge?" The nurse, with fifteen years' experience on him, sounded skeptical. I was content to stare at the ceiling, wishing I could scratch my nose. The rest of their back-and-forth floated past me like smoke. I picked out only the words I wanted to hear, the ones, finally, that meant my part was done: I slumped against the wall and peeled off my gloves. They talked on. The patient snored. With any luck I could be home by dinner.

Early the next morning I was back, studying the numbers

the Swann had generated. They filled up Marie's flow sheet. On the floor, where vital signs are checked perhaps once a shift, a patient's flow sheet can fit a week's records to a page. On the Unit, a single day's sheet is a foldout thirty-four inches long, a grid with boxes dedicated to every physical parameter of human existence. Marie's that day was dark with ink.

The section I was studying held numbers that were supposed to reveal Marie's fate: cardiac output, cardiac index, left ventricular end-diastolic pressure, systemic vascular resistance. These were why we had put her through that exercise, but as I scanned the numbers back and forth, they told me nothing.

Not that I am an expert in the interpretation of Swann-Ganz catheter readings. We were getting into territory where I was clearly little more than a collector of information. But I knew enough to see that the numbers we were getting didn't add up. If, three weeks into this rotation, I still knew how to add. If I still knew how to care.

"We see this sometimes," the attending explained. "In the end stage everything just falls apart."

"But what does it mean?" the fellow asked, waving the flow sheet. I was gratified to hear confusion in his voice, too.

The attending shrugged. "It means she's falling apart. The physiology just isn't there anymore."

There was a long silence, during which the stately puffing of a ventilator in a nearby room became more and more distinct.

"So what's keeping her alive?" I asked.

The attending turned to look at me. "Nothing," she said flatly.

I HAVE A CLEAR MEMORY from this period, although what day exactly this might have happened I no longer recall, of the attending emerging from Marie's room and stopping to brush at her eye before sitting to write in the chart. I remember it so vividly, like something glimpsed from a speeding train, because at the time it had no meaning. I could make no sense of it. It may not have happened at all. After three weeks of q3 call, dream and memory had become indistinct, the one unwelcome as a distraction from sleep, the other unwelcome always, the dead and discharged claiming time beyond any I had to give.

The next day we were on call again, the cycle starting to feel unbearably compressed. When the PA announced a code at the start of rounds we ran, but it was a sore, hobbling kind of progress we made, Alex and the intern and the medical student and I traversing the length of the hospital and up the old main stairwell to 5 West, where we found the usual melee in progress. Owing to our slow pace on the stairs (at the fourth floor we stopped running), the MICU team had gotten there first. From the doorway, over the crowd of nurses, techs, and assorted hysterics, I couldn't even see the patient: just the rhythmic up-and-down of whoever was doing compressions. The MICU team waved us off. We walked slowly back to the CCU.

Marie's room was crowded when we reached it on our rounds, three or four figures gathered at the bedside, their backs screening her from us as we stood outside the door. At a glance they were clearly nonmedical, probably family, and I tried to shut the door before I presented her, but after thirty years the doors in the CCU do not close. So I presented the data on Marie in a low monotone that no one but the attending could hear. No one else was paying much attention, the fellow and Alex fiddling with the radiology monitors, the intern slumped in her morning fog, the med student staring at his clipboard as though it held portents of his own impending death. There was little to report. Her ins and outs had been barely negative overnight, and her creatinine continued to climb. The Swann numbers were a random sprinkling of figures that I reported without conviction. As I trailed off, the attending simply shook her head, and swept into the room.

A laugh was ringing through the air as we intruded on the bedside, the sound of it bouncing unnervingly loud off the walls. A woman at Marie's right elbow straightened, pushing back a stray curl, and smiled at us, a bright, airline hostess's smile. She turned to Marie.

"Your doctors are here, honey. We'll just be going along."

"I'd like you to stay," the attending said, and turned to Marie. "We need to have a conversation."

Marie, floating in the bed like some enormous whipped dessert, gestured weakly at the two women at her sides. From somewhere on the peripheries, a pale, balding man wearing a failed comb-over and muted checked trousers shyly waved.

"Have you met my girls?" Marie asked.

"Not yet," the attending said, holding out a hand to the

one nearest, the one who had called Marie "honey." "I'm Dr.
Sparrow," she said.

"Jeanine Wright." She took the hand and they held hands
briefly. "We're her girls." The woman at the opposite elbow
nodded assent, but her gaze remained on Marie, a fixed,
mournful expression I had seen before.

"Do you need us for something?" Jeanine said.

The attending, her lips thin, nodded. "I think Marie may."
She turned. "Marie."

Marie looked up at her from the bed, the tremor that always
inhabited her jowls momentarily quite pronounced and then
still.

"How do you feel?"

Marie gazed back at the attending. For a long moment the
two of them looked at each other.

Her voice came out with a husky sound. "Like it's time to
go, Doctor."

The attending nodded. She reached out and took Marie's
hand. "Do you need more people to come?"

Marie heaved her gaze around toward the mournful woman
on her left. "Did you talk to David?"

The sad eyes lifted. "He said he'd be here tonight."

"And Ralphie?"

"Tomorrow."

Marie settled back, shifted around to the attending. "Do I
have tomorrow?"

The attending lifted Marie's hand slightly, moved it gently
side to side, then set it back down. "I think so."

Marie subsided into the bed. "I'll be here," she said, and

then her voice rose in a thin husk of a laugh. "If I'm not anywhere else."

The girls at her elbows laughed too, bright bell-like voices breaking out of them, washing over us in our rumpled whites in a wave of human sound.

The code that morning seemed to have disturbed the rhythm of the day. The emergency room was quiet for once, the cath lab down for maintenance. The whirlwind of admitting fell strangely still. I had time to see my patients.

I left her for last, skipping over the alcoholic cardiomyopathy whose snores were audible from the door.

Her girls were still there when I entered, the two of them bending over the bed (the bed itself raised to elbow height because Marie, as she had observed, wasn't getting out of it, and the nurses prefer not to stoop). The checked trousers were cross-legged in the room's sole chair, nodding pleasantly at me as I entered.

"Doctor," Marie said, as I came around the foot of the bed. "Have you met my girls?"

I held out my hand to Jeanine, who took it in a brief, soft clasp, then reached across the bed to the quiet one. "Francie," she murmured, an apologetic smile. Her eyes were red.

Jeanine turned to Marie. "We met your doctors this morning, remember?"

"Not this one," she said. "He's the quiet one." She turned to me and her jowls creased in a conspiratorial smile. "Aren't you?"

"I suppose so," I said, suddenly very shy.

Marie turned to her girls. "This is the one I was telling you about. My morning buddy. Aren't you?" The same sly grin. "He's the one comes in to squeeze my knee."

The girls tittered. I could feel heat spreading over my face.

Jeanine, clearly the responsible one in the party, shushed her. "You're embarrassing him, Mother."

Marie peered at me. "Why, honey, you're right. I never dreamed doctors could blush."

Jeanine attempted to rescue the situation. "Mother says you're very nice."

A distinct pain stung me, centered in no anatomical structure I could specify. "Your mom's been nice, too," I replied.

We all stood there. Thinking about the tense I'd just assigned Marie, no doubt.

"She's been telling us how hard you all have been working."

Marie stirred, a proprietorial pride in her voice. "This one never sleeps."

The girls made clucking noises as Marie expanded. "I see him out there all hours of the day and night. The nurses tell me he has a family, but I don't think he ever sees them. Do you?"

"Do you have a family, Doctor?" Jeanine asked. I nodded. Additional questioning elicited the snapshots I kept in my pocket. Marie reached out an eager hand.

"Oh, they're beautiful boys," she cooed. "Look at that one, Jeanine. He looks just like Roger. Doesn't he look like Roger, Francie, when he was little? Right down to the drool on the chin." Uproarious laughter, and I realized Roger was the name of the checked trousers. "Come here, Roger, and tell us if this little boy doesn't look like you." Roger, shyer even than I, joined us at the bedside. "What's his name, Doctor?" Marie asked.

There is a boundary I don't cross over with patients. I don't mind showing pictures of my kids: over and above the fact that I'm fond of my children, I've found that showing their pictures can humanize an otherwise awful situation. It's useful. But I don't tell their names. It's a privacy issue, basic protection of hearth and home. But there's also a primal superstition at work. Naming calls. To use the names of my children in the CCU would somehow connect them to this world and what goes on here. That's where I draw the line.

But not that day. I told Marie their names, the names I withhold from this account, and she made the appropriate sounds, repeating them, identifying each in turn. The girls agreed they were sweet boys, and their names were lovely names. From which point it was impossible to proceed with the conversation I had come in to hold: just when and how Marie should die. But I proceeded anyway.

These things must be done delicately. This was a point the attending had underscored for me earlier that day, when she had reminded me that under no circumstances was I to switch off Marie's dobutamine until I was certain she was past feeling. "The minute you turn that off, you know what's going to happen to her, don't you?"

I started to give the right answer, but this wasn't one of those quizzes.

"She'll drown," the attending went on. "You don't want her to be aware of that."

We had reached the point of discussing the morphine drip.

"Morphine drip" is really more of an expression. It's not often that you actually have a patient getting a continuous infusion of IV morphine. But we use the expression anyway, to signify the crossing of a threshold. We were about to put Marie on a morphine drip: we were about to make good and certain that, as she died, she would not suffer.

I remember crossing a street in a European city years ago, when a pigeon fluttered to the pavement after colliding with a car. It flopped helplessly for a moment, something clearly very wrong with it. Without breaking stride, a man stooped in the crosswalk, seized the pigeon in one hand, and with a quick twist stopped its fluttering. He set it back down and walked on. I remember most clearly the expression on the man's face: a mask, concealing what? I remember also that he held his hands away from his sides as he went on. No doubt he washed them not long after.

Modern medicine cannot—thank God—administer that quick twist. The only way to save Marie from feeling that long fluttering was morphine. But my attending was instructing me that it had to be done carefully because morphine, while it masks the sensation of suffocating, also suppresses respiratory drive. And so it has to be done carefully. If at all possible, it should be her heart failure that kills her—not our attempt to save her from suffering.

None of this, of course, entered into my conversation with Marie and her girls. Despite its impossibility, the discussion went off well enough. I hemmed and hawed, then explained what we could do to honor Marie's request. They listened to me with a respect that always unnerves me, nodding solemnly as I stepped them through what I thought Marie might need. When I was done, I looked at her. She was lying there with the washed-out look of someone who has in fact quit fighting. "What you think best," was all she said.

Two hours later I checked back. Marie had absorbed two milligrams of morphine, a dose that does more to sedate than cut pain, which was fine. She needed to get some of it ahead of time, to feel it working in her and know what it was. More family were there. They drew me into the room, by some Brownian kinetics of handshake and question pulling me toward the head of her bed.

"Here he is," I heard her say. The morphine had, paradoxically, livened her up a little. She was propped in bed, keeping court. As I was drawn into her orbit, the crowd parted and fell in behind me. "Here's my doctor," she said proudly. "Jeanine, tell him what we were just talking about." She dimpled deeply, and Jeanine explained, "We were talking about her ice-cream cone. It's a story we tell." A general murmur, the laugh we give in appreciation of a long-loved joke, welled behind me.

I did my part, looking puzzled, prepared to be amused.

Jeanine started. "One day, years ago—"

"It was the year after Mother died," Marie explained quietly.

"Yes. It was Easter. And Granddaddy took Momma and Aunt Ellie and Aunt Peg out for ice cream." Jeanine paused, looking to Marie to take up the prompt.

"He promised us if we didn't fuss in church we'd all get ice cream."

Jeanine smiled. "After church, he bought each girl an ice-cream cone. And then he set them out on a bench in the park across the street."

"He wanted a picture of us in our Easter dresses," Marie said, coming in so quickly she almost cut Jeanine off. Her voice had taken on an authority I'd never heard there. "And he wouldn't let us start to lick until he took the picture. They were starting to drip, but he wanted a picture before our faces got all messy. He had a Brownie camera that was always difficult for him, unfolding it and all the settings. We sat there wanting to lick our cones and so afraid they were going to drip and spoil our dresses." She stopped, winded. The expression on her face was intent but turned inward, concentrating on her breathing, or pursuing something in the story she could not quite recall.

"And then, just as he was about to take the picture," Jeanine prompted, "just as he said to the girls, 'Say "Ice cream—"'"

"We all said, 'Ice cream!'" Marie's face lit up with the words. "But just then—" She caught her breath. We all caught our breath.

"Out of a clear blue sky . . ." Jeanine whispered.

Marie shook her head as if a fly had touched her face. "The most enormous wind came up, and whirled around us so hard it seemed it would pick us all up into the sky."

Jeanine, Francie, and even Roger were all leaning forward, intent on the figure in the bed, and as Marie's pallid jaws worked I could see the rest of them moving their lips in unison.

"And when the wind blew away . . ." Jeanine began.

"When the wind died," Marie continued, "Mary Ellen had

her ice cream." The silent chorus echoed, *Ice cream.* "And Marguerite had her ice cream." We were all of us leaning toward her. "But when I looked at my ice cream, it was gone! My ice-cream cone was empty!"

We stirred, the spell on the verge of breaking, sharing looks in a ritual of amazement in which I, too, was included.

"We looked and looked, on the bench and in the grass, in my dress and even in my little pocketbook, but no matter where we looked—no ice cream!"

Marie's eyes were shining now.

"And then," Jeanine prompted one more time, "Grandaddy said . . ."

"Daddy said," Marie began, her eyes softening, turning inward again.

"Granddaddy said," Jeanine repeated as Marie faltered, "'Don't worry, Marie, God sent that wind to blow that ice cream up to heaven.' And Momma said, 'Daddy, that don't make sense. There's all the ice cream they need up in heaven!'"

The ritual wound up in an outburst of gaiety, but Marie, wattles quivering with indignation, shook her head. The outburst died.

"That's not what he said."

Jeanine and the others stared at her, stricken.

"I know that's how Mary Ellen liked to tell it, Jeanine, but I was there. What he said was, 'The good Lord knows where your ice cream went, Marie, but I sure don't.'"

She clamped her jaws together and glared at nothing in particular.

Out of the awkward silence, Francie's voice rose.

"What happened to the photograph?"

We all looked at her. Defensively, she added, "I've always wondered. If Granddaddy was taking their picture, wouldn't that show where the ice cream went?"

We all turned to Marie, who shook her head again.

"Daddy said when he went to rewind that film something went wrong. The sun got in and spoiled the whole roll. Every negative came out as black as black."

"No picture?" Francie asked plaintively.

Marie's expression softened. "No, Francie," she said quietly. "There never was any picture."

"And your ice cream?"

Marie, looking inward again, said almost inaudibly, "No ice cream, either."

THAT EVENING, I LOOKED in briefly, but the room was quiet, Marie asleep, one of the girls slumped half over the bed. The monitor high over Marie was the only sign of life, the green light dancing in the darkened room. She was restless, her face twitching, brow furrowed, but still she seemed asleep. Dreaming, I thought, then pushed the thought away. I stopped at the nursing station to order two more milligrams of morphine.

In the morning, after rounds, after another sleepless night, I went in to shut off Marie's dobutamine. Her pressure had started drifting down, but otherwise there had been no change. The whole family had gathered again at the bedside, joined by a few more faces that shared the stamp of Marie's pointed chin and broad forehead. There was also a large, freshly bathed and shaved figure introduced as the pastor. It was time.

I went to the head of the bed. Marie looked up at me. "Hello, Doctor," she said.

"How are you?" I asked, the question sounding less inane than I expected it would.

She waved a hand vaguely. "Here," she gasped, attempting a laugh, and then the hand subsided.

"I'm going to turn off the dobutamine now. Is that all right?"

"Yes. Turn it off." She almost rose from the bed with a sudden vehemence that startled me.

"Are you sure?" I asked reflexively.

"Yes." Her voice rose sharply. "Turn it off. Now!" With her left arm she gripped my sleeve. "You promised."

She was wandering, I thought, addled by morphine and fatigue, drifting in and out of a place she did not trust. I only nodded, and turned to the nurse who had quietly followed me in. She bent beside the IV pole. The pump sighed to a halt, the grinding noise that had been unnoticeable up until then suddenly loud in its absence.

Nothing changed. The family stood still, looking at Marie as if they expected her to expire on the spot.

I moved back to the bed. "There," I said.

She looked at me.

"Are you okay?" I smoothed a curl back from her forehead.

"Fine now," she said. And then her right arm reached around and gripped my shoulder, pulling me toward her. I bent, obediently, thinking she wanted to say something.

Instead she planted a dry kiss on my cheek. I hung there a

moment, holding my breath. Then I kissed her back. The skin of her cheek was very cool. She sighed, and her grip relaxed. I turned and left the room.

It took Marie four hours to die. I was in and out of the room, checking for signs of distress. There were none. On one of those visits, I reached up and turned off the bedside monitor: she had a pacemaker, and I didn't want the family to see the tracings continue after she was dead.

Around three-thirty, the nurse found me at the station.

"Twelve is gone."

I sighed, and pulled myself upright.

MARIE'S BODY: THE FACE gone slack and chalky, the eyes blank; her lips, half open, expressionless. Within her chest I heard nothing. A fugitive creak and gurgle as fluids shifted in her, but the heart itself was still. Time of death was 3:32. Cause of death, congestive heart failure. I filled out the papers as quickly as I could.

"DOCTOR?"

I looked up, focusing with difficulty. It was Jeanine. Her eyes were red, mascara smeared across both cheeks.

"Marie wanted me to tell you."

"What?"

"Two things. She said to thank you. And that she knows where that ice-cream cone went."

I waited.

She shook her head. "That was all she said. 'Tell that doctor I know where the ice cream went.'"

I looked at her and she shrugged, smiling.

I smiled back and we parted, hugging each other in the decorous way strangers should.

LATER THAT DAY, FINALLY, I went home. I lay awake a long time that night, in the desperate insomnia that seizes me sometimes, post-call. I was thinking about that ice-cream cone, wondering what Marie had meant, what revelation had come to her as her brain, starved for oxygen, fogged with drugs, had started to shut down. I have seen it before. My own father, dying on a morphine drip, his kidneys gone from a failed dobutamine tune-up, had spoken in his last coma. Stray words. Words I hung on through the long afternoons. I no longer remember them.

Where could that ice-cream cone have gone? It had fallen somewhere they hadn't thought to look. Everybody in the room, all of them sharing that story over all those years, must have known it. That wasn't the point, though. But then what was? I tortured the question for a long time, as my wife stirred beside me in her sleep, and one of the children murmured something over the carrier hum of the baby monitor, and nothing came to me. Just ice cream, Marie's finale, the long slide downward into night.

That night I dreamed. I have found that picture. Deep in it, the figures move, the three little girls in their neat white dresses throwing up their arms and shrieking silently as the wind whirls, leaves and debris fly around them, and in the distance trees thrash their limbs against a glaring sky. I scan the picture, searching it for a dim white blur ascending, flying skyward out of the frame. That night and three times since I have dreamt this, and each time I awake into the dull non-knowledge that I have failed to find the ice cream. I know that one day in this dream I will learn where the ice cream has gone, where Marie has gone, where all of us will someday vanish, ice under the sun. Unaware that this is but the dream still upon me, I watch helplessly as it recedes into the light, whirled upward on a wind that leaves me cold and dark and dumb.

THE
SURGICAL
MASK

ἐγώ εἰμι ὁ ὤν

T HE REFERRAL HAD COME IN THE DAY BEFORE. Richard, the on-call nurse, had jotted down a sketchy story: Sylvia Turner, a fifty-seven-year-old woman being discharged from Memorial after treatment for a sinus infection. I looked up from the form at the duty nurse with whom I was rounding that morning. "Sinus infection?" I said. "Is that really an indication for hospice?"

Linda laughed. "Is that what he wrote down? Give me that." She took the referral from my hand and swiveled it around. "That idiot." She laughed. "He left out the part about the cancer. Squamous," she added, and tapped the side of her nose.

"Ah," I said, meaning I was sorry for Mrs. Turner. Like leprosy, only worse, runaway squamous-cell cancer whittles its victims away until the tumor reaches something vital to life, and then they die. "Anything else about her?"

"Husband says she's stopped eating."

"Is that a problem?" I asked. With hospice patients, when they stop eating it's usually a good thing.

Linda shrugged. "That's where Richard ran out of info. She's first on the list, however," she added brightly. "Shall we go ask her?" She hoisted her red backpack and stomped out the door. Linda, I had learned, despite the impression she gave of having spent the weekend playing electric guitar in a goth band, was a highly reliable if somewhat profane nurse. In my four days so far with the hospice team I had also learned to follow her obediently from house to house.

My presence on the hospice service was an elective month, one of two my residency program permitted. Hospice had looked promising because: (a) it got me out of the hospital, and (b) I didn't have to come in on weekends. And, I had told myself, it would be a relief to work with patients whose deaths were welcome.

I spent the drive in a pleasant half doze as Linda drove. I suppose if I'd paid attention to her driving I'd have been less relaxed, but in this, as with her dispensing of morphine and laxatives, I was content to let her steer.

I know now that much of this passivity was simply evasion. It hadn't taken many visits to homes where death had become part of the décor before I started to think that in electing a month of hospice I'd possibly overdone it. But it was only a month, I told myself; if I had learned nothing else from residency so far, it was that I could do anything for a month. So I did what I'd learned to do very early on in my training: pull in the antennae, lean back, and watch the scenery go by.

Which it did, in an alarming series of loops and swerves, until we scattered gravel in front of a rambling one-story farmhouse standing in the midst of a rain-soaked yard. The sparse lawn was broken by a barely graveled arc on which we had come to rest beside a large gray pickup truck loaded with what appeared to be chicken coops. An old fruit tree, thrawn with age and neglect, dripped rainwater across a faint trace of bricks that marked the approach to a swaybacked porch.

Linda, muttering as she backed the Accord into a vacant patch of gravel, scanned the yard and surrounding outbuildings. The back of the house seemed to abut on an overgrown orchard. Linda surveyed this suspiciously for a minute. "Don't see any," she announced finally. She was talking about dogs, which she had explained to me our first morning were the only thing she really worried about on these visits. She had illustrated this by displaying a large, crescent-shaped scar on one calf. I followed her to the porch, hunching my shoulders to keep the rain off my neck.

On the screen door a handmade sign, black marker on a sheet of cardboard, read *No Visitors*. Behind the screen, the door stood slightly ajar; it bore another handmade sign with the same message. As we stood looking at the signs, the door opened abruptly, framing a very large man in a faded flannel shirt, with a round face and pale curly hair fading to bald on top. He eyed us warily.

"Hospice," Linda called through the screen, a jaunty singsong, two notes, descending. She showed him her backpack as if it explained our mission.

A weary look of relief broke through the suspicion. "Sorry about the sign," he said as he backed out of the doorway. "We had trouble yesterday."

"What sort of trouble?" Linda was already in, peering

around the darkened interior like a bird looking for something to peck.

"Some ladies from our church." He fell silent for a moment and I could see the muscles of his jaw knot suddenly. "They wanted to tell Sylvie how she's going to Hell."

"Shit," said Linda.

Mr. Turner nodded once emphatically. For a moment he looked as though he was about to cry.

"Is she okay?"

He glanced reflexively into the darkened interior. "She had a bad night."

"Could we see her?" She shouldered her pack, then caught herself, held out a hand, and made introductions.

He took her hand, looked over his shoulder at me. "Charles Turner," he said gruffly. "Thanks for coming." He turned toward the interior. "She's in here."

He led us down a dim hallway, and as my eyes adjusted to the interior murk I was startled: under a ceiling at least twelve feet high every wall was filled with paintings. Not reproductions, I realized: oils on canvas, framed and hung one above another from the chair rail to the pressed-tin ceiling. Landscapes, most of them, graceful imitations of Constable; some were portraits after Reynolds. They were beautifully executed: solemn, Academy-quality exercises in every way, except that in almost every one the classical landscape was disrupted by the presence of large tropical birds: scarlet macaws, cockatiels, lovebirds, flocks of parakeets. In the portraits, birds perched on shoulders, peered coyly from behind the sitters' heads, or preened on outstretched fingers, the sitters gazing lovingly.

Massed above us in the darkened hallway, their effect was slightly hallucinatory.

Turner paused as we stared upward. "I framed them," he said quietly.

We looked at him.

"They're Sylvie's," he added, surprised at our obtuseness.

He led us through a doorway at the end of the hall. We entered a dining room, which by the clutter everywhere had not been used for dining in a long time. A battered mahogany table, chairs and sideboard cowered beneath canvases depicting enormous parrots; these were minimalist, primary-color cartoons on a stark white ground. We moved on to another low hallway. At the far end, a half-light door let out onto what looked like a chicken house: wire cages and roosts, rustling forms, an occasional muted screech. Turner led us through another door and there was the bedroom.

The curtains were drawn. The dim light of the rainy day outside barely illuminated the canvases that lined each high wall: a kitchen table in sunlight, large earthenware bowls with birds roosting on their rims; a picnic after Manet, the figures holding out crackers toward the trees; a tropical waterfall with small pink forms that I realized after a moment's confusion were human infants, winged, fluttering through the mist. In the surrounding trees, enormous cockatoos were sheltering untidy nests, from which more small human faces peeped. In a queen-sized bed Sylvia Turner lay, shrouded by a flesh-colored chenille spread. She had watched us come into the room: her eyes—large, liquid, and brown—had followed us as we entered, and I'd been aware of them on us as we stopped and took in the display on the walls. Her expression as we gazed upward was hard to read.

I'd had the impression that the bedspread had been pulled up almost to her eyes, but as I stopped staring, finally, at the paintings and turned to the bed (where Linda was already bending over, her hand out to take Sylvia's), I saw that what I had mistaken for part of the bedspread was a surgical mask covering the lower half of her face. It ballooned slightly in rhythm with the rise and fall of her chest; it fluttered when she spoke. It muffled her voice as she said something in reply to Linda's questions about her pain, or I thought it did, and then I realized her voice was simply indistinct, as if speaking around a mouthful of pebbles, the consonants slurred or reduced to soundless puffs into the mask.

It was the sound of her voice that made me look at her.

She looked back, the eyes shrinking from mine at first, then coming back to meet my gaze a moment, then sheering away.

I continued to stare. There was nothing there but a surgical mask, no sign of anything unusual about it at all, except that it was overlarge: the edges lapped over her ears, the ties barely visible as they extended around her head and neck. Just a large white surgical mask. I could barely keep my eyes off of it.

I realized Linda was speaking to me.

"She says the Roxanol isn't working."

I nodded, still struck mute at the mask fluttering in and out.

"Roxanol," I said stupidly. Roxanol is an old brand name for a concentrated elixir of morphine, the mainstay of hospice care. No IV needed: just a drop or two under the tongue and it's absorbed.

"I think maybe she's not absorbing." Linda bent and whispered something. The eyes closed briefly as the head bobbed once on the pillow. Guttural noises whispered back into the nurse's ear.

Linda straightened abruptly as if recoiling, caught herself, and walked around the bed to my side to speak confidentially.

"She says her tongue's pretty much gone." She paused, suppressing something I could not read in her face, then added, so softly and fast I almost couldn't catch it, "Most of it sloughed off a few nights ago."

I stared at her.

"That's why she's not eating."

I didn't know what to say.

"Say something," she hissed, nudging me with one elbow. She gestured with her head toward the face on the pillow.

"Mrs. Turner?" I said as I edged toward it. "I'm Dr. Harper." I stopped at the head of the bed. The mask fluttered, but no sound came out.

I reached out and took her hand. She let me, let it rise off the bedspread as I went through the motions of taking her pulse. This is something they teach you in medical school: when you don't know what else to do, check the pulse. It breaks the ice.

Her pulse was on the rapid side, and not very vigorous. Looking at her eyes, I suspected she was dehydrated.

"Are you in a lot of pain?"

The eyes closed. Then opened again, as she nodded. Without the lower half of her face, it was hard to read her expression.

"How much pain?"

She stared at me for a long moment before she shrugged.

The combination of her mask and her silence, the economy of her gestures, the dullness of her skin in the gray light, all made her seem more like something carved in marble than human.

"Do you think you're swallowing the morphine?"

Another nod.

This time, I nodded back. "You'll need a higher dose," I said.

The eyes above the mask were looking at me. I had a brief, vivid impression that what she was really doing was measuring me for a canvas, a parrot on my shoulder.

I shook the thought away, disturbed by it more than I wanted to be, chased it away with an overly detailed explanation of how we were going to treat her pain. I moved on from there to her difficulty swallowing. I had figured out by now, looking at the profile revealed each time she inhaled (the mask fluttering in to cling against the face), that there could be no nose left under there. There seemed, in fact, to be a cavity. And then I realized where I had heard that strange pattern of lost consonants before: in children with a congenitally absent palate.

I kept trying to imagine, to construct a clear picture of what her oral cavity must be like, but I could not come up with an image, just shards of what I might glimpse if I pulled away her mask. I tried to puzzle out how the cancer could have spread from the roof of her mouth to erode the root of her tongue when a voice behind me made me start.

"She's not eating,"

I had forgotten the husband. Charles Turner loomed out of the shadows, his voice a rumble in the dark.

"I can't get her to take anything." The rumble twisted slightly at the end, caught on the last syllable.

The figure on the bed lifted a hand. It hovered, palm outward, brushing gently at the air.

"Sylvie—" The voice was half a plea.

The eyes closed and then the hand made one last sweep, waving us away.

IN THE DINING ROOM, the parrots gazed down on us as we sat at the table.

Linda laid her hand on Turner's hairy paw.

He turned toward her, reluctantly met her gaze.

"What do you think she wants now?" Linda asked.

"I think she wants—a nap." He shook his head and blinked repeatedly.

Linda looked at him for a moment, then nodded.

"That's right," she said. "I think she's tired. And when she rests, maybe you can rest, too." With a glance at me she reached to the floor and pulled her backpack into her lap. I leaned back and let the conversation go on without me as Linda counted out on the tabletop a boxful of syringes filled with pink syrup. The parrots watched silently.

A booted foot caught my right shin. "Isn't that right?" Linda was saying brightly, looking at me with an expression that didn't match her voice.

"Yes," I said automatically.

She rolled her eyes and turned back to Turner. He hunched

in his seat, his large hands holding a handful of syringes like
a lover's posy.

Linda kept talking to him gently. "So we think it makes
sense to treat it," she was saying.

Turner looked up, smiled at her faintly. "Thank you," he
husked. The parrots hunched motionlessly, as if waiting for
something.

Outside, the rain was coming down harder, spattering the
windshield as Linda pulled the wheel around. She was looking
at me instead of the road.

"What the hell got into you?"

"What are you talking about?"

"You just checked out in there." She pulled out onto the
pavement. I watched wet woods slide by and let the silence
grow. I had nothing to say.

"Sometimes," Linda said finally, "something about a case
can be too much for you. It happens to everyone. It helps if
you do your job anyway."

"What are you talking about?" I said again.

"You didn't even examine her."

That stopped me.

She was right. I'd stood there by the bedside, taken her
irrelevant pulse, and talked about drug absorption and swallowing, her fluid status, and at this point I couldn't remember what else, but hadn't done the simplest thing to assess
the situation.

Which would have been lifting up that mask and seeing
what lay beneath.

"You're right," I said.

Sometimes I find myself in a situation so confusing that the only thing to do is tell the truth, I think.

ONE OF THE ESSENTIAL skills in residency is a capacity to forget. There are some things you just don't want to take home. I had no special facility at this skill, but I was usually able to set aside whatever needed setting and pick it up again the next day. The hospice rotation had been no different in this regard: whatever tragic or pathetic or sordid or horrific scenes I passed through each day faded like dreams before I reached home.

Which is why I was disturbed, that night as sleep evaded me, to find Sylvia Turner's face looking out at me from the darkness, the eyes above the blank white mask. I had learned not to remember faces. I had learned not to be disturbed. I wasn't bothered (I thought) that her face—the absence of it, whatever it was that white mask implied—was disturbing; I was bothered that it was still visible to me at all.

If I was frightened by its persistence, by the possibility that it was asking a question of me, I mistook my fear for annoyance. But even if I had recognized what I felt, I could not have told you what it was I feared. There was just the blank square covering—what?—and that was more than enough.

THIS VAGUE SENSE OF annoyance was gone by Monday. I dozed through morning staff meeting, through updates on who had died over the weekend, who had been doing badly, who needed to be seen today.

Linda nudged me with her elbow. Arthur, who had been on call over the weekend, was looking at us.

"What happened?" Linda had just asked, a little too brightly, overdoing it in a way that I felt dimly as a reflection on me.

Arthur's expression went cloudy. "I'm still not exactly sure." He riffled his notes. "The husband called, about twelve-thirty Sunday. P.m.," he added fussily, looking over his glasses. "About some 'church ladies' he wanted off the premises."

"And what did you do, Artie?" Linda asked innocently.

"About church ladies?"

Dry laughter rustled in the corner.

"I mean, were they . . ." Linda paused as if searching for a word. "Causing a disturbance?" She was clearly enjoying herself. Everyone else was laughing.

Arthur was reddening. "As a matter of fact, they were," he replied. He read without expression, "Patient's husband reports 'Church ladies are back again,' and upsetting patient with unwanted religious advice. Husband wants church ladies removed and sedation for patient."

He looked up again over a hedge of paper. In the overhead fluorescents, his glasses had taken on an opaque glare. "I offered to call the sheriff, and reminded him about the Ativan in the comfort pack. I think what he really wanted was the Ativan."

"Don't we all," somebody muttered, stirring laughter again.

"THOSE CHURCH LADIES ARE going to ruin our day," Linda growled, spinning the Honda's front tires in the hospice lot. She pulled out onto the highway thirty yards in front of an oncoming gravel truck. I closed my eyes. "Ordinarily," she explained, "the Turners wouldn't be on the list again until Wednesday." She straightened out the wheel and gunned the engine. I settled back to ignore the ride.

The day was bright, the air cool, still drenched with last week's rain. Puddles stood in the gravel arc before the house, reflecting patches of pale sky. The reflections shivered in the breeze.

The house itself might have been deserted. From somewhere out back rose a strangled cry—for a brief moment it seemed the sound of someone calling for help, and then I realized it was a parrot. It called again.

"Bah!" it seemed to say. Then, more clearly, "Bad!"

Linda looked at me. "Do you think that's one of the church ladies?"

"Bad!" the bird called again. "Bad! Bad!" Linda's joke, and the repeated screeching, combined to set my skin crawling: I thought of a small, angry old woman crammed into a wooden hutch, screaming.

"Listen," she said, cocking her head.

"Bad bird!" the parrot called. Then, after a pause that stretched out as if in contemplation, "Go to hell!"

Linda burst out laughing. "Who trains a bird to talk like that?"

Charles Turner was waiting in the doorway, looking slightly embarrassed. "You heard that," he said.

"What, the bird?" Linda laughed again. "Hard to miss it."

He smiled weakly. "Sometimes we get calls from the neighbors." He glanced back over his shoulder.

"Just let the bird tell them to go to Hell," Linda suggested brightly.

"He's not the one the neighbors complain about." Shaking his head, he led us down the hall.

"What do you suppose the other birds say?" Linda whispered to me. By the time we had made our way through the darkened dining room, I realized I was hunching my shoulders, prepared to fend off a verbal assault. But no more sound came from the back of the house.

In the bedroom, Sylvia Turner sat propped up on pillows. The mask fluttered, puffing out a series of nonsense sounds.

I had a chilly moment wrestling with the possibility that the words really were nonsense, Mrs. Turner driven mad by whatever the church ladies had said. Then Linda started to laugh.

"You didn't teach him that?"

Mrs. Turner rolled her eyes heavenward.

Her husband, still standing at our backs, said quickly, "Lord, no. They're rescued birds. They came that way."

Another burst of sound from Mrs. Turner—a string of vowels, low and flat.

Linda laughed again, but though I listened closely to the mangled words I couldn't put them together.

Shaking off a sadness that irritated me for being ungrounded in anything I could name, I moved to the bedside opposite Linda.

"Mrs. Turner?"

The mask turned toward me. The eyes were unreadable. Had I interrupted? Off in the distance, a bird was croaking something about a pretty girl.

"We heard you had some trouble yesterday." I said this as gently as I could, but still it felt like I was pushing something faster than it wanted to go. I was anxious, I realized, to get out of there.

And while I was trying to penetrate the jungle that had grown up in my own motivations, the woman on the bed started to cry.

It took me a while to recognize this. What I saw, from my perspective, was initially obscure. The face above the mask simply crumpled, withdrew, eyes squeezed tight. Then, after a sharp intake of breath, the mask plastered itself against the lower half of her face: as it clung there, it showed for a distinct instant the outline of a crater far too large to belong in any human face. It reminded me of the plaster casts archaeologists make of the voids left where something has crumbled into rust. Then the mask bulged out again on a gust of inarticulate woe. The face turned away from me, burying itself in the pillow, where, twice muffled in cancer and down, it sobbed. I watched her shoulders heave, how clearly the bones slid beneath skin. This woman is starving, I thought.

Linda's hand appeared, stroking the lank hair. A movement at my elbow caught my eye, and I gave way to Turner as he bent over the bed. He was muttering something I could not catch beyond a tone of barely contained rage. At me? I wondered momentarily. In the distance, a parrot uttered an obscenity. Turner glanced up in that direction, straightened, and in a very low voice repeated it. The room fell still, the word rolling through the stillness like thunder far away. From the pillow, muffled but clear, the voice spoke what it could of the man's first name, a short *a* cut off at either end, but the tenderness and the mild reproof were clear enough.

The big man glanced around sheepishly. "I'm sorry, Sylvie," he said.

She straightened, but kept her gaze to herself as she tugged at her hair; some wisps had stuck to the fabric of the mask, held there by the tears that had soaked into it. She pulled the hairs away, composed herself, smoothing the spread. "A," she said again calmly, and then something more. Turner's face clouded again.

"They can too help themselves, Sylvie. They just don't want to. They—" He broke off. "They're just vultures," he growled, and fell silent again.

Sylvia rolled her eyes. The gesture looked very odd from where I stood: without a face to support it, the expression lost its moorings, as if her eyes had gotten free from their sockets and in the next moment might fall onto the pillow. She closed them briefly, as if drawing them back in. When she spoke again the tone was a determined contradiction.

Turner snorted. "'Christian,' my eye."

Sylvia nodded emphatically.

"What has 'Christian' done for us lately?" Turner snarled, turning away.

For a long moment, Sylvia's gaze lay inscrutably on her husband's back, and then the head turned back to the pillow, and from its depths came again the sound of muffled sobs.

This time they did not subside. As none of us said a word they began to rise in pitch and volume. From the distance a bird took up the cry, inarticulate screeching now. Another joined in. The birds sounded distressed—or was the tone, too, only mockery? The crying on the bed grew louder, one clawed hand reached out, clenched the pillow, withdrew, formed a fist, and began pounding on the bed. With each blow the cries grew louder, higher, and from the end of the house the screeches of agitated birds came back—echoes, I kept imagining, of Hell. Harpies, I was thinking. Or was it Furies? I couldn't remember which was which, I realized, as the shadows of Linda and Mr. Turner moved in, hovering over the bed.

SOME TIME LATER, after the Ativan had done its work and Sylvia had subsided into sleep, the three of us sat around the dining table. Linda had been trying to think of some means of fending off the church ladies. The hospice chaplain, she thought, could call them. Turner had refused, shaking the suggestion off as a horse shies flies. In the awkward pause that followed, Linda pointed at the wall.

"Is that you?" she asked. It was clear she was trying to change the subject, giving Turner a ladder out of the dark hole he had dug himself into.

Turner looked up, laughed bashfully. "Yeah."

Linda let out a bright peal. "Did you pose for that?"

Turner shook his head emphatically. He was coloring up to his receding hairline. I turned and craned my neck. It was clear which of the canvases she meant: a large oil of a muscular male nude standing in a hubcap emerging from the sea.

Hovering at the figure's shoulders, a pair of scarlet macaws clutched in their beaks the ends of a long leather tool belt, which looped between them in front of the figure, obscuring its genitals but little else. The figure gazed modestly toward the shallows; in the air above it, flights of cockatoos flushed pink in the sunrise.

We all gazed at it for a while.

"She loved to paint," Turner said quietly.

"Yes," Linda said. "I can see that."

Turner brightened. "It shows, doesn't it? How she just loved it? And the birds—" He twisted away. "She loved everything." There was a long silence. I could hear a faint metallic twanging from the back of the house. When he spoke again his voice was barely audible. "She used to love everything," he said.

Linda reached across the table. "She still does."

He did not look up. "I don't know," he said quietly. When he looked up again, it was to study the wall. "I don't know what I'm going to do with these."

"YOU DID GOOD IN there," Linda said as the farmhouse receded behind us.

I stared at her. Was she joking?

When I did not respond, she gave me a sidelong glance. "Bringing up those church ladies," she explained.

Had I done that? How that had helped anything I could not begin to fathom.

"All I did was make her cry," I said.

"Exactly."

I puzzled over this until she added impatiently, "We're *hospice.*"

"Oh."

"She's dying: she needs to cry." The tires thumped and she pulled the car abruptly onto the shoulder. "*He* needs to cry." She stared meditatively out the windshield. "I'm not sure I want to be around when he does."

"Ah," I said.

Another sidelong glance. "'*Ah?*' Are you getting this?"

"Oh, yeah," I said. "I get it."

She stared at me flatly for a long moment, until I grew embarrassed and turned to look out the window.

WHEN MY SON WAS not quite four, he had drawn a picture that was supposed to represent a spleen, a swarm of red and purple dots he had copied laboriously from a textbook on histology. His teacher had been so charmed by the description ("spleen, mag 240x") that she had taken it off that afternoon to an art show put on by the hospital, children's drawings meant to brighten the lobby. From which it had never, tragically, returned. The disbelief, then anger, and finally inconsolable sorrow, had lasted the better part of a week. They still resurfaced months later, a muted echo wistfully raised at odd moments, from the back seat of the car, or twenty minutes after bedtime, to which my own and my wife's helpless response had become almost automatic. But we also felt a trace of that same sorrow, not so much from the loss as our helplessness in the face of it.

My sleep that night was broken repeatedly by that helplessness—dreams, fragments of nightmares in which lost things cried plaintively out of the dark. But when I went to find them there were only drawings of whatever it was I so urgently sought: crude, parodic cartoons, mocking my deep need. And even as I held each crumpled bit of drawing paper, the voice kept crying, somewhere else.

LEAVING U.S. 1, WE descended into a wilderness of wooded hollows, surfacing into small clearings of abandoned tobacco holdings, then woods again, until we stopped in a crunch of gravel. A small cabin perched at the edge of a four- or five-acre clearing, much of it fallow and ragged with early weeds, but around the house a neat plot of fescue lay smooth and emerald green. The cabin looked vaguely like a chalet, the clapboard siding pine under varnish. Inside, the walls and kitchen cupboards were all the same yellow pine, shining dully in the morning light. The front room was dominated by a large picture window, and directly beneath it a low single bed, on which lay a man who might have been sleeping, but his eyes were open, fixed on the view outside. He gave no sign that he heard us enter, ushered in by a small woman in a brilliant purple dress. She brought us back into the kitchen, where she steered us to the long pine table.

On the wall by the sink a framed rotogravure showed Jesus on his knees, praying beneath a lowering purple sky. Facing Jesus from the other side of the sink was a yellow sunflower woven from colored straw. It bore the rubric, *Every day is a sunny day somewhere.* The image of Jesus did not bear this out.

"Doctor?"

The woman was looking at me, evidently waiting for a response. Off to one side I saw Linda looking amused.

"I'm sorry," I said. "I didn't catch that."

"That's all right, Doctor," the old woman said. "You've always got a lot on your mind, I know." She settled herself in the other chair. "I was just saying it was so good of you to come."

There was something here, as well, that seemed to be saying more than I could grasp. She sounded almost as if I had been here before and she had been expecting me to return. I looked around the room, half hoping to find some clue, but the more I looked about the kitchen, the more firmly it refused recognition.

Until my gaze fell on the refrigerator, where, among snapshots of a diverse assortment of young people, half of whom had been caught in the process of graduating from middle school, I saw a sheet of bright yellow paper (the same shade as the sunflower still trying to cheer up Jesus by the sink) headed with a red stop sign: a standard out-of-hospital DNR form. There, at the bottom of the form, was printed my own name, and below it my illegible, unmistakable signature. I had met this woman before. And the passive figure lying out in the front room: I knew him now. Terminal heart failure, discharged to home with hospice. I had taken care of him in the hospital two or three months before. Alston: the name came back to me at last.

I cleared my throat. "How is he?" I said.

The woman looked into the front room, intent for a long moment on the figure on the bed. Then she looked back at me.

"He's not good, Doctor." Her voice was flat, her expression unreadable.

Finding myself here, so unexpectedly, in a home I had never thought to enter (one of the inescapable facts of hospital medicine is that, upon discharge, a patient vanishes from sight), I felt as if my presence here was a falsehood. This woman thought I had come to see how her husband was. She thought I had remembered him.

How many patients had I discharged this way, I wondered, patients I knew were going home to die, and never had a moment to think of again? I couldn't begin to guess, no more than I could count all the others who had died in-house: for a long moment I saw a flickering of images like a primitive newsreel: not their faces, not their names, just shapes in beds. I could remember much better the rooms in which they had spent their final hours, sometimes multiple ghosts inhabiting the same room: their rooms, their diagnoses, and sometimes (these were the worst), when I could remember faces, it was only how they had looked when I had come into the room to pronounce them dead: the blank mask where before had been a personality.

I looked around at the bright, spotless kitchen, the woman's face across the table still expressionless, and my presence in this house seemed the inevitable outcome of all those unthinking discharges: I was here to expiate some sin of omission.

I had just begun to contemplate how little I knew about the expiation of sin when Mrs. Alston shook her head.

"He's not good, Doctor," she said again. Then, dropping her voice, in a tone that combined urgency and grief: "Why didn't anyone tell us what it would be like?"

I felt a stab of guilt.

Linda was at her shoulder, murmuring something I couldn't catch. Looking over the woman's head at me, she gestured toward the front room: "Go see Mr. Alston," she said. I rose and left the kitchen, relieved to be anywhere else.

The figure on the bed shifted as I came in. Mr. Alston's face seemed inscrutable at a distance, but as I approached and the eyes followed me, I recognized what it held: the utter weariness of a man whose heart had failed. When we had discharged him, he had been too weak to lift himself from his bed; if I had thought about it I would have given him only a week or two. But he was still here, his heart still feebly beating, the chest still rising and falling, the minutes continuing to pass and each day following the last into the night. He watched as I approached, as impassively as I imagined he watched for Death itself, because his life had narrowed down to this: watching or not. The eyes followed my approach, but beyond registering my existence they gave away nothing.

"Mr. Alston?"

The eyelids closed.

"Are you all right?"

The absurdity of the question felt like a slap in the face, but he gave no sign, and for a moment I felt a surge of anger: What else was I supposed to say?

"Is there anything . . ."

I wasn't sure what I wanted to know.

"Is there anything you want?" I finished lamely.

The eyes opened. A hand appeared from beneath the quilt and grabbed my arm. It pulled me down, the strength in it shocking, until I was close enough to smell the decay in his mouth. For a long moment he held me there, the eyes searching my face. Then he gave the slightest shake of his head and turned away. I wasn't sure if he was answering my question or dismissing me, pronouncing judgment.

The two women both looked up as I reentered the room.

"How is he?" Linda asked, her studied cheeriness deflecting any questions. As I muttered something bland and noncommittal, I realized suddenly that Linda, for all the time I had spent in her company, was almost as much a blank to me as Mr. Alston. If I had noticed this before, I would have said this was her nursing training, the professional polish that kept her work from consuming her, but now I was unsure. Perhaps she seemed that way only to me. Perhaps I really understood nothing, nothing at all. I looked around the kitchen, and the room, for all its sunny cleanliness, seemed as inscrutable as if it were the work of an ancient civilization. In the portrait of Jesus, the bruise-colored sky looked sinister, Gethsemane just one more episode in an endless history of suffering. A history from which I wanted only to be excused.

"Thank you, Doctor," Mrs. Alston said.

I could only stare at her.

"For coming," she explained. She rose from the table, levering herself up to her full five-foot-one, and made her way over to me in a series of short, rolling steps. She slipped her warm, dry hand into mine and gave it a tremulous squeeze.

"Doctor," she said quietly, and her voice had a note in it beyond sadness, an unmistakable tone of the reproach I always worry I will hear. "Doctor," she said again, and squeezed my hand one more time, using it to turn me back toward the front room. We stood and looked together at Mr. Alston gazing out the window. She whispered, "Why didn't you tell me that it would take so long?"

WEDNESDAY MORNING, AS I followed Linda to her car, she asked, "Ready for a trip to the bird museum?"

After a few moments, she asked again.

"You up for it this morning?"

"What?"

"The Turners," she said, sounding a little exasperated. "Are you going to show up this time?"

The car swooned around a turn that tightened as it curved, and for a dizzying moment I thought we might skid, but Linda's grip on the wheel didn't shift; we hit the straight. In that moment I had experienced an inner equivalent of a near-skid: I saw the past week and a half of this rotation as they must have looked from some other perspective. I had been a shadow, a cardboard cutout, the mere image of a man, through the whole thing.

Linda was still looking at me.

"I don't know," I said.

THE GRAVEL PATCH IN front of the Turner house was occupied. Two cars—large, middle-aged sedans, one a tan Buick, the other a dark blue Olds—were parked nose-to-nose beside the old fruit tree, which in the past several days had pushed out plump buds frilled with pink. The sun was working on the last of the morning haze, heating everything to a silver shimmer. As we pulled onto the gravel and Linda killed the engine, I thought I heard the parrots screaming.

"Uh-oh," Linda said quietly.

Above the voices of the birds a dark rumble rose, breaking into deep, staccato barks. For another moment I allowed myself to believe a dog had gotten in among the birds—a vivid flash of red, green, yellow swirling feathers flying, shrieks of outrage, inhuman voices shrieking "Bad dog! Bad dog!" The image was frightening enough: my heart hammering high in my chest, I stared at Linda for a cue.

Linda stood half out of the car, looking not toward the back of the house but over the tops of the parked cars toward the porch. The Buick blocked my view, but, even so, as I tried to follow Linda's gaze I realized the sounds weren't coming from the back of the house. And then what I thought was barking resolved into a man's voice, shouting a single obscenity over and over, overwhelming a chorus of high-pitched protests that sounded now less like "Bad dog," and more like "Praise God." Or perhaps I was only forcing sense into what was actually inarticulate shrieking.

Certainly by the time Linda and I rounded the rear bumper

of the Olds and stopped, separated by five or six yards from the knot of figures on Turner's front porch, the sounds coming from the group had broken down entirely into shrieks and wails, broken repeatedly by Turner, who stood filling his doorway, red-faced, the muscles and veins of his neck standing out like the anatomy of Hell. Which was what he was saying now to the group of women surrounding him: *You go to Hell! You go to Hell!* He said this more times than I wanted to count, the words taking on an incantatory force, as if he expected his rage to blow an opening in the air.

He advanced, one straight-legged stagger, then another, the porch shuddering at each *Hell!* as his feet came down. The women were wearing, I realized, Sunday churchgoing dresses. Several of them clutched small Bibles at their chests, like shields against the assault; others held their hands to their ears and turned their faces sidelong away and down, their own mouths open in Os of dismay. The whole scene had a weirdly static quality, like a medieval landscape with figures, a saint or a prophet, a hostile mob. I waited for someone to pick up a stone.

Linda struck out for the porch, her backpack over one shoulder, passing through the knot of church ladies as though oblivious to them. She took the two steps in one stride to Turner's side, her hand out to rest on his forearm.

He shied it off, staring pop-eyed at her as if unable to make sense of what he saw: a slight, pale figure in black leather amid the dark purple proprieties assaulting him. He blinked and turned back to the crowd, seeming to mouth one last invocation of *Hell!* but his voice made no sound. His mouth opening and closing would have been comical if the whole scene hadn't been so entirely terrifying.

What have we walked in on? I started to turn away, in what should have been the prelude to a quick retreat. But Linda and the keys to the Honda were on the porch beside a red-faced lunatic, in the middle of a circle of strange women who seemed to be gathering themselves, now that Turner had fallen silent, for a new assault.

What have I gotten myself into? I got no answer. I tried a few tentative steps toward joining Linda on the porch. Not that her position seemed any more secure than mine: I only followed some avian instinct to flock in the face of danger. In the relative quiet, my footsteps were loud in the gravel; here and there heads turned.

Are you going to show up? Linda's question came back to me with a different inflection. But before I could imagine how I might answer it differently, Linda's voice—cool, neutral, smooth as water—broke what had become almost a silence: even the caged birds behind the house, I realized, had fallen still.

"Hey, Mr. Turner," she said. "What's going on?"

She might have intended this as an innocent question, but the church ladies, choosing to hear it as a general inquiry, sent up aggrieved cries, crows wheeling above a stubble field. The gabble conveyed nothing articulate, only a sense of outrage and violation, trailing off into a single woman's voice muttering, "Thinks he knows who's going to Hell . . ."

Linda held out both hands, making shushing noises.

"Ladies, ladies," she said. "I'm from"— I could see her switch gears in midsentence—"the hospital," she announced, in tones that stressed the institutional bulk of "hospital." "And this—" She brightened, as if in enjoyment of some inspiration. "This is the doctor from the hospital." Her outstretched hands moved to indicate me, catching me on the steps, where I had frozen when the outcry broke out. I may actually have waved, weakly, to the faces around me.

"We're here to see our patient," Linda explained. "And we're going to have to ask you"—she turned her gesture into gentle shooings—"to leave now. Our patient needs quiet. The doctor"—she turned a beneficent smile my way—"needs . . . to examine her. Isn't that right Doctor? You're going to examine her?"

The performance was working: at the invocation of hospitals and doctoring, at the specter of something as improper as a doctor's examination, the ladies backed out of their semicircle, the flock breaking up into scattered knots and muttering. I couldn't help wondering, even as I registered overwhelming relief, if Linda's question to me had been more than theatrics: *You're going to examine her.*

Was I? Shaking myself as if emerging from deep water, I climbed the steps and crossed the porch, past Turner (who seemed also to be awakening from a spell), into the darkened hallway.

I knew the way: down the hall, through the dining room, another hall (where pale pink cockatiels perched frozen in the limbs of steel-blue trees), into the bedroom, where light suffused through drawn shades, and a slight figure marked the otherwise blank rectangle of the bed, the head a smudge on the oblong pillow, and in the midst of the smudge a white square.

Her eyes, half obscured by the mask, were looking back at me, a long, expressionless inspection.

I looked up at the wall, anywhere but at the face on the bed. Before me hung a series of miniatures under the rubric *Life Cycle of the Hyacinth Macaw*: it began with a clutch of pale tan eggs and ended with a single large blue bird, the eye in the center of its golden ring peering directly out of the frame, a knowing smile on its beak.

What did it have to smile about?

"Ey ih or eh-er."

Her voice was soft, as if some small creature perched upon my shoulder had whispered in my ear. Startled, I turned toward Mrs. Turner. She had turned, half raised herself on one elbow. She was watching me look at her paintings.

"Ey. *Ih*. Or *eh*-er."

"'They live'?"

She nodded.

"'Forever'?"

I must have sounded skeptical. She shrugged. "Ong ime. Eh chur ee."

"*A century?*"

She nodded, but her face above the mask was as blank as her own short future.

"Is it smiling?" I asked suddenly.

She nodded again.

"*Can* they smile?"

Another shrug.

I crouched beside her for a moment. I realized I was looking at the mask again. As I looked, it billowed gently toward me. I drew back.

A cold hand on the back of mine caught me. I forced myself to look.

"Arh oo a rai uh ee?"

The tone was quiet, and try as I might I could find no accusation in it. But her eyes were pleading.

"Afraid of you?"

The eyelids dipped.

"No," I said reflexively, my tone a protest.

She looked away.

"No," I said again, much more quietly, leaning closer to her. The lie was palpable in the air between us. But how could I bring myself to say I was afraid of her? How cruel was that? In a doctor, how cowardly? She seemed about to cry again. I heard myself say, "No. I'm not afraid of you."

The hand rose from the bed, dismissing what I'd said, and I knew in a moment it would be waving me away as well.

"I'm afraid of what's happening to you," I said, the words tumbling out of me. "I'm afraid of what will happen to you. I'm—"

The hand rose again, but instead of dismissing me the fingers brushed across my lips. The touch of them was electric. To this day I still feel it.

"Ohn orry a'out ee." She swept her hand before her, embracing the room, the pictures, the house. The gesture ended in a half wave toward the window, where I could hear a car starting up, gravel crunching under tires. "Orry a'out all 'ih."

Beyond the doorway, somewhere in the house I heard a parrot scream. And as if in answer from another direction I could hear the rising sounds of a man sobbing, sobs bursting into deep howls of grief. Her eyes cut to mine, the eyebrows rose, and her hand compelled me toward the door.

Quiet sounds followed me from the bed. Her last words were unintelligible.

In the kitchen, Turner sat slumped at the table, shoulders heaving as he sobbed. Linda, patting his back, looked up as I entered. *She okay?* she mouthed. I nodded. She looked at me another moment, her gaze briefly intent. *You okay?*

I thought before I nodded, and took a chair on the other side of Turner's heaving form. I did not try to pat his back. But I sat there until he was done crying, and when he straightened, his face shining, and started to apologize, I heard myself make a low shushing sound.

"Don't worry about it," I said.

Back in the car, Linda gave me a sidelong glance.

"What?" I said, more irritably than I intended.

"Well?"

"Well what?"

"Did you examine her?"

"Yes," I said.

"And?"

"She's fine."

A few days later, the morning report began with the news from the on-call nurse that Mrs. Turner had died around eleven p.m. It had been peaceful. Services would be at Siloam Baptist at three on Sunday.

I sat stunned in my seat, doubly so because even as the thought of her death refused to make sense, I was puzzled to find myself so affected. *Hospice,* I said to myself. *People die.* Had I learned nothing?

I shook my head involuntarily. Linda, at my side, was looking at me.

You okay? she mouthed.

I thought about this again, before I shrugged. She nodded and turned back to the meeting.

As the meeting broke up and Linda shouldered her pack, she said to me over her shoulder, "You going?"

I thought about the Turners, and myself, and hospice one last time.

"Of course," I said.

THE AFTERNOON WAS HOT for the time of year, the sun harsh on the raw red clay, the green shade under the awning inadequate for the gathering at the graveside. I tried to recognize the church ladies who had been in Turner's dooryard the week before, but in the crowd the dresses and hats and hairnets and dour expressions were impossible to distinguish. I held back as the preacher read his text, not really following, letting the murmur of the eulogy, the Jesus and the sins, the clay and the dust, the resurrection and the hope eternal all fade into the larger stillness of the late Spring afternoon.

White stones shimmered in the heat. A bluebird perched atop one, distinct amid the shimmering. At intervals it dropped to the ground, returning with something clutched in its beak. Beyond the churchyard, massed loblollies and poplars kept their shade to themselves. In the distance, a wren was scolding; a crow barked as a smaller bird harried it over the treetops; high overhead a trio of turkey buzzards teetered on the air. As I looked and listened, the stillness of the day came gradually alive with birds. They were everywhere.

I found them wherever I looked—a thrasher rustling dead leaves under azaleas; a mockingbird flipping its tail from the low branches of a dogwood; sparrows hopping in the dust— and told myself that Mrs. Turner's fascination with birds had been a testimony to something in her I had never had a chance to see, an appreciation for the life around her. The idea was comforting; it was probably not much different from whatever the preacher was saying.

Whatever the preacher was saying, he was done. There was a long, dreadful pause, and then the static arrangement of the mourners began to dissolve, currents of dark suits and dresses dispersing among the graves toward the parking lot. I watched a while longer. I had spotted Linda earlier, among the group of mourners just outside the awning. I waited for her to emerge, passing the time observing how the birds receded from the human tide: I thought I could see them watching from the higher branches of the trees, waiting for the last mourners to cede the churchyard back to them.

I could see Linda speaking to the large, balding figure of Charles Turner, the two of them nodding and bobbing back and forth. Then Linda turned and pointed in my direction, Turner looked as well, and the two of them began to make their way from the grave toward me. As they approached, I could see that Linda had worn a navy blue dress, in which she was almost unrecognizable. Turner, too, in a business suit seemed as out of place as a robin in a cage. He carried a parcel, a rectangle done up in brown paper and twine. Linda carried another like it.

"Doc," Turner said quietly. He extended his free hand, then the one with the parcel, and for a moment neither one of us knew what to do until Linda laughed. Turner shook his head as if shying off flies. He thrust the package at me again: "Sylvie wanted you all to have these."

I stammered something, looked to Linda for an explanation, but all I got was a shrug. I took the parcel, the hard ridge of the frame under the paper telling me what I had already known.

"Is it one of hers?" I asked, knowing the question was stupid.

Turner nodded. "She thought you should have it." He looked away for a moment, out over the roof of the church, and cleared his throat. "She painted these after she got sick."

I stood there, at a loss for words.

"Open it," Linda said.

It was an oil on canvas, a portrait of an anonymous young woman posed against some indefinite outdoor space, the sky pale blue beyond her head and shoulders, a bright, suffused light filling the frame. She had light brown hair that fell in ringlets around her neck. Her eyes were open wide, her mouth an O of delight as she looked up to her side. Her right hand was lifted as well, index finger extended; a moment ago it had been the perch of the bird that now hovered, wings uplifted at the top of their stroke, the object of her gaze. It was a parakeet, pale blue, almost the same color as the sky, so that it seemed to be fading into the light that lit the woman's face. Then I noticed the bird had a tiny, distinct golden halo over its head. And that the woman's head, too, had the faintest suggestion of a halo as well. Linda's painting could have been its twin, except in hers there was no bird at all, only the same faint glory over the same rapt skyward gaze.

"I can't take this—" I began.

"She told me to give it to you, Doc. One to Linda and one to you." He looked at us, his red-rimmed eyes giving us a direct stare, the force of it almost palpable. "I've got a thousand others. And if I had a million more it wouldn't—" He broke off. "I don't need it."

"Thank you," Linda said. She was signaling me with some message I didn't get. I was stammering, and then the three of us fell silent again. Somewhere the harsh call of a jay refused the silence.

"Thank you," I said finally. We looked at the paintings a moment longer. The face in each was lovely. I wondered if Mrs. Turner's face had once been so luminously beautiful, or if, behind her mask, she had felt free to paint something other than she had before.

I would never know.

WHEN I GOT HOME, I left the painting in the garage until after the children were in bed. I brought it in then, and for a long time my wife and I looked at it. "It's a beautiful painting," she said.

For a long time afterward, whenever I closed my eyes, I would see that painting shimmer indistinctly in the darkness. When I opened them it still hovered, a vague shape drawing nearer, ghostly, a faint rectangle of light. As it approached it would resolve, and finally reveal that face now hidden in the undying darkness of the grave.

IRON
MAIDEN

THE HOSPITAL WAS A TERRIFYING PLACE TO look at. A fortress of weather-stained limestone, it glowered over the surrounding city from its hilltop, surrounded by oak trees that had been old when Sherman's forces had marched by. Seen at night during an electrical storm, it completely fulfilled whatever fantasy the words "psychiatric hospital" might conjure. But the ancient oaks, the gray-streaked limestone, and the razor wire were only superficial aspects of a building that had, within its walls, four-hundred-plus patients whose appearance was anything but terrifying. "Sad" was the word that came most often to mind.

On the ward for which I was responsible, there were on most nights three or four dozen women, ranging in age from their late teens to their early sixties, hospitalized for treatment of their substance abuse, depression, mania, suicidality— a profound inability to get along with the rest of the world. Most stayed only a week or two, cycling between the ward and the streets, returning sometimes after as little as six or seven hours outside the walls. On each admission, each patient had a physical exam and medical history taken by the psych intern. On Friday and Saturday nights, my first responsibility as the medical moonlighter on call was to review these new admissions to the acute women's ward.

I was grateful to have the job. In the final months of my training, anything that eked out the salary I earned as a subspecialty resident was welcome. Here I earned a dollar a minute and went home at midnight. The work wasn't heavy, consisting primarily of overseeing the intern, and often it was interesting, from a medical perspective. The patients had a startling variety of medical illnesses.

As for their mental illnesses, especially once the acute manifestations had been bottled up, this was generally a drab affair. The patients lacked much in the way of facial expression, their clothing had a similar threadbare quality, and their histories tended, through repetition if nothing else, to have rubbed off all the corners that might once have made them the distinct stories of individuals. After so much cocaine, prostitution, and cutting of wrists, after so many delusional pregnancies and divine possessions, in the strong solvents of alcohol, street life, and psychosis, individuality dissolves.

On my first night I arrived still wearing a necktie. The nurse who met me in the medical unit laughed out loud. "Best take that off, hon," she said. This struck me as dramatizing, but I complied. And although in certain areas of the hospital (the forensic wing, chiefly) it seemed only a fool would give anyone a handle to grab hold of, among most of the patients one felt not fear so much as a guilty aversion, a continual, if muted, grating on some inner nerve, the emotional equivalent of someone dragging heavy metal furniture across concrete several floors overhead.

Each evening, after letting myself through the two sets of locked doors that sealed off Acute Women's, I couldn't get halfway to the nursing station before patients would start to flock around me, all of them talking. Some wanted to tell me about a symptom they were having, or show me some unusual sign. More often it was a plea for discharge (in which decisions, thankfully, I had no say). Sometimes it was to adjudicate disputes with another patient, a nurse, a doctor, a parole board or judge, or some personality I could only hope was imaginary. Occasionally I was met with a flat stare, or accused in ringing tones of terrible crimes. I walked quickly, avoiding eye contact as much as I could.

Most nights there would be only three or four admissions to review, and in most cases my contribution was nothing more than a quick summation of the intern's findings and a listing of the key points of the medical plan. Whenever the intern's note suggested anything worrisome, however, it was part of my responsibility to repeat the history and physical.

In that environment, knowing what to worry about and what to ignore was sometimes hard. As historians, the patients were not unreliable so much as inscrutable. When a woman tells you she has a baby in her finger that's one thing; but when she tells you she feels crushing pressure in her chest every time she climbs the stairs *without* a towel around her head, that's another. These were patients capable of hiding, behind the fog and mirrors of madness, all manner of disease.

For all my worries, whatever I felt called on to investigate turned out usually to be straightforward: the patient had come in with a fever, or the admission labs had revealed some metabolic derangement, or there had been a complaint elicited on history like fainting spells or a recent assault. If the intern had been busy, or the patient less than cooperative, these things might have escaped a workup. Occasionally something subtler would catch my eye: some inconsistency in the history, usually, that would start me worrying. And sometimes it was just a hunch. I'm not a fan of hunches, generally: too often they're shorthand for a diagnostic process being rushed. But in a psychiatric hospital it seemed inevitable that decision-making should hinge on the shadowy unnamed.

It was one of those shades of doubt that led me to pull Carrie B back off the stack of papers I had reviewed. She had been the third of five admitted overnight, and the one after her, with HIV and hepatitis C, a fever and abdominal pain, had consumed an hour of my time, during which the intern had been paging me repeatedly from the floor, where his handling of a series of emergencies ranging from constipation on Gero to a scalp laceration on Acute Men's required my oversight and approval. And I had ordered a pizza, which was by now getting cold at the reception desk. But something about Carrie B bothered me, and I pulled her sheaf of papers off the stack for another reading.

As charts went, hers was nothing special. In her previous admissions, she had been too healthy to warrant much in the way of medical attention; the bulk of her chart was devoted to psychiatric treatment, in which I generally took little interest beyond noting the primary diagnosis. Her prior admissions had been for self-injury and borderline personality disorder. Now she was back again for the same thing: a few slices at the volar surface of her left wrist, too superficial (in the intern's assessment) to warrant suturing, which is usually the case in the ones that survive.

None of this accounted for the anxiety her account set roaming in my chest. What had gotten my attention was something else: the description in the "General" section of the physical exam. This usually consists of the rote *WDWNWF, A&Ox3, NAD* (for "a well-developed, well-nourished white female, alert and oriented to person, place, and time, in no apparent distress"). For Carrie B the intern had taken the time to interpolate a relatively prolix *uncomfortable-appearing*. She had also exhibited pain with deep inspiration, as well as with palpation of the liver. I considered the relatively brief list of what could cause such things. There had been no prolonged travel or immobilization suggestive of clots migrating from legs to lungs, no recent trauma or motor vehicle collisions, no report of an alcoholic binge; vital signs were unremarkable; urine pregnancy test was negative. Her admission blood work was still in the lab.

Without having actually laid eyes on her, I knew uncomfortable, pleuritic, tender-livered Carrie B might be harboring any of a dozen different processes that could carry her off by sunrise Sunday: but it seemed unlikely. More probably she was (as the expression has it) "responding to internal stimuli." This is a phrase psychiatrists love. "Responding to internal stimuli" means the patient is hallucinating. It's a way of characterizing crazy behavior that sounds more clinical than it is. Only a crazy person responds to internal stimuli. But she had no history of psychosis. She was simply a borderline.

Borderline personality disorder, I had learned in medical school, like all personality disorders, occupies a gray area between the transient disturbances common to us all and the major diseases of mood or cognition. This gray terrain is not the borderline the term refers to, however. People carrying this diagnosis predictably lead lives of chaotic instability, alternately attaching to and breaking from, with equal violence, the people around them. Everyone with whom they have to do for more than a few hours they either idealize or demonize. Craving attention, they are said to suffer from a deficient sense of self. Asked how they feel when they're alone, generally they'll say, "Empty." The border they inhabit is the one between having a personality and not.

None of this qualifies as psychotic. Sometimes borderlines will produce symptoms simply for the attention, but outright shamming is usually reserved for highly specific, tactical maneuvers: chest pain on the day of discharge, for instance. The need for attention runs deep; they prefer actual physical disease to simulation: hence the self-injury. Whatever was bothering Carrie B seemed to me more likely physical than delusional. But the presentation was so vague, it could be anything. Had she been assaulted? Was she harboring a broken rib? A collapsed lung? Had she swallowed something? Was her gallbladder going bad?

I leaned to the gallbladder. It was an explanation I liked for several reasons: it was probable, it was not alarming (medically or spiritually), and the workup was relatively straightforward. But there were all those other things that needed ruling out. With a brief pang about the pizza cooling on the reception desk, I shoved the chart back in the rack and asked the charge nurse if she could bring Ms. B to the examining room.

The examining room was a closet off the common room. Its door, like every other door in the facility, was kept locked, separating the patients from the needles and knives, alcohol and iodine they would be better off without. Having the master key, I could have let myself in and waited while the nurse fetched Carrie B, but I am just claustrophobic enough that I preferred to wait outside.

Which meant I had to wait in the common room, where the same women who had mobbed me on entering the ward now milled around, waiting for the distribution of evening meds, watching television, or simply milling. In this environment, standing motionless conferred a small measure of protection against direct importunities. To be still and quiet in that setting was to make oneself practically invisible.

I stood against the wall and watched. A dozen women, dressed in pajamas, sweat suits, or oversized hospital gowns worn as a drab sort of muumuu, were gathered restlessly before the locked Dutch door of the medication room. The rest were watching, more or less, the television, which from its bracket high on the opposite wall emitted a nearly continuous series of deep-chested thuds. A car rolled over and burst into flames, bringing a loud cheer from a group on the sofa, when the nurse rounded the corner with Carrie B in tow.

Even across the common room she was visibly uncomfortable. She walked as though made of something thin and brittle. When the group on the sofa hooted, she flinched, but even in flinching she held her upper body rigid.

In the examining room, with the nurse's assistance she climbed carefully onto the table, bracing herself on her arms as she sat on one end. Looking up from the chart, I identified myself. She looked at me, her features thin and pinched, her gaze a little too direct. There was a pause, during which she sniffed once or twice, and shifted uncomfortably on her perch.

I attempted a disarming smile. "I wanted to find out how you're feeling."

She sniffed again, then carefully extended her left arm in my direction, and rotated it slowly to bring the bandage at her wrist into view.

I looked, but did not move closer to inspect. "Does it hurt?"

She looked at it curiously. "No." The arm hovered in the space between us, quivering slightly before—slowly—it withdrew.

When Carrie B was done with this languid demonstration of her capacity to hurt herself, there seemed little more to say. I recalled—with an effort—that it wasn't her wrist I was worried about. I'd never entertained the possibility that her presentation had anything to do with the superficial lacerations on her wrist. Like any good stage magician, she had waved her hand in front of me knowing that it would distract me—knowing as well that it would hold my attention on her.

But tonight the show was plumbing some new depth

of drama. What was going on in Carrie B that held her so uncomfortably on the edge of the examining table?

"Would you mind lying down?" I held up the bell of my stethoscope. "I'd like to listen to your heart."

She made a face, a brief curl of her lips as if she had tasted something unpleasant, and then began to lower her upper body to the surface of the table.

It was an extraordinary performance. Her hands, which had been braced on either side of her, walked haltingly back toward the head of the table, while, inch by inch, she levered her body down. Her face took on a series of different expressions as she moved: eyes opening wide, as though astonished by something, then wincing, then widening again, her pupils very large in a way that suggested some huge autonomic discharge to which I was only a peripheral witness. She caught her breath repeatedly, in a series of gasps, each cut short. As she settled the last six inches I found my own breath catching in my throat.

As her back touched the table, the three of us—the nurse had been holding her breath too—let out a long sigh. I glanced over my shoulder at the nurse, who was looking back at me, her RN's deadpan broken to the extent of an elevated eyebrow. Shaking my head, I leaned over Carrie B and placed my stethoscope on her chest.

A healthy young heart thudded under my hand. Air moved freely as she breathed. Her respirations were rapid and shallow, and her pulse was rapid as well. Moving down to her belly, I let my stethoscope lie there for half a minute, listening to the ordinary gurgling of an untroubled digestion. Then I started bearing down on the bell. This is an old trick: if you suspect someone is overreacting (as many do) to overt pressure, but fails to respond to the more subtle pressure from the stethoscope, you can be fairly certain that their reaction has more to do with mental processes than abdominal ones. But I hadn't gotten more than an inch or two down before I heard a sudden sharp intake of breath, followed by a spasmodic clenching of the obliques.

I looked at the patient's face: it was pinched, pale, except for two distinct red spots over her cheeks. Her eyes were closed, and her breathing fast and shallow. I listened again, and heard only the subterranean gurglings of an ordinary belly.

Tentatively, I placed a hand on the right upper quadrant, fingertips two inches below the margin of her ribs. "Take a deep breath," I said, and prepared to dig in to find the edge of her liver. As she started to comply, her breath caught: her eyes flew open again with the same odd expression of surprise, and wild, dilated pupils. And something else: behind the surprise something kept close.

I lifted my hand from her belly.

"Does that hurt?"

The gaze she turned on me was theatrically blank.

"What?"

"When you take a deep breath. It seems to hurt you."

"Oh. Yeah." Pause. A tentative trial of deep breathing, staged carefully up to the point of pain. "It does. A little." She smiled at me then, and there was nothing stagy about the smile, and there seemed nothing duplicitous about it, either: it was actually a very nice smile, winning, even, and I thought for a moment that Carrie B might under other circumstances have had a pleasant life. Instead of being not much short of terrifying. I looked back at her, trying to get her to come into focus: a small woman with finely chiseled features, pale blond hair with a slightly reddish cast to it, and it struck me that she was unusually well groomed. Her hair was clean, her skin clear, although I knew the color on her cheeks was more hectic than health. All of which was only a setting for the disturbing thing that glimmered in the depths.

"Do you think it's anything serious?" she asked.

"What?" I said, a little abruptly. I muttered something non-committal, as I always do, and started to scribble orders in the chart. There was a staginess in the question I found irritating. I hadn't time for it. My pager was going off again, cutting like an alarm clock through the fog that had filled the room. The nurse picked up her clipboard in a gesture so matter-of-fact it seemed staged as well. Was everything staged? I wondered briefly, one of those odd thoughts that surface all the time but took on too much meaning in a place like this. "Frequent vitals," I muttered, and left the two of them to manage as best they could. I finished up my orders—X-rays of the chest, expedited—and left the chart on the unit clerk's desk.

THE PAGE THAT HAD broken the spell in the examining room had been the intern, who was waiting for me outside the second set of locked doors. He had a somewhat hectic expression himself, a shock of thick black hair standing straight up from above his forehead. As he read off from his clipboard summaries of the three cases he had already seen and the seven more that were waiting, he repeatedly brought his hand up to his forehead and drew it back across the top of his skull. He seemed to be trying to press it—the top of his skull, not the crest of hair—into place, but the only effect was to make the crest stand even higher. That, and the way his eyes kept opening very wide, made him look a little mad himself.

I couldn't blame him; as he dutifully read off the minutiae marshaled on his list, I had the impression the nurses had been leading him on a merry chase around the building. Half of what he had been called about was, as usual, junk. In a medical hospital they wouldn't have merited a note in the chart, much less a page to the on-call MD. But here the staff didn't have the luxury of deciding what to ignore: they were required to call for anything out of the ordinary, and did. And the intern was required to see everything he was called about, no matter how unlikely. And now that I was done reviewing admissions, it was my job to supervise him as he made his rounds.

The intern—his name was Joe Bellagio—was one I had worked with several times before, and every time it had been like this: so busy we barely had time to talk about anything beyond the exigencies of the case at hand. I hardly knew him, beyond an impression of a tall, skinny fellow who usually seemed more rattled than he actually was, who took his responsibilities seriously, and generally knew what he was doing. He seemed sensible, thoughtful, and kind. All of which inclined me to like him.

He reached the end of his list of pending calls. "Who needs to be seen most?" I asked.

He studied the list again. "I think the guy in F-Max."

"The chest pain?"

"Forty-eight, diabetes, smoker, eight out of ten for the last"—he checked his watch—"thirty minutes." He checked his list. "And a prior MI."

My own heart bounced slightly on a passing wave. "F-Max, huh?"

"Yeah."

I sighed. "It's chest pain." And stopped. "Can't they send him over?"

Joe was walking at my side, head down, hands thrust in the pockets of his lab coat so his elbows stuck out behind him. He shook his head without looking up. The gesture made him look like a discouraged stork.

"Can't do that anymore. Not from F-Max." He glanced at me. "There was an incident."

We had reached the front lobby. My dinner, the white cardboard box going a translucent brown along the edges, was sitting on the counter at reception. I scooped it up as we passed. The guard looked up from his screen, said, "It's cold by now," and pressed the button that let us out.

The night outside was loud with crickets and katydids, the humidity thick enough to scatter the glare of the sodium vapor lamps over everything. Objects stood out with a weird vividness, wearing halos in the streetlight. As we crossed the parking lot, a raft of palmetto bugs froze at our feet, then scattered madly in all directions. We watched them vanish. The slice of pizza I had been stuffing in my mouth had lost some of its savor. I gulped it down anyway.

"There's a metaphor," Joe said quietly.

This was not the kind of thing I usually hear from interns, even in psychiatry. I offered Joe the open pizza box. "A metaphor? For what?"

He shook his head. "Not sure." We started walking again. As we turned out of the parking lot into the darker street, he said, "I think it's for our relationship with this place."

He gave me a sidelong, self-conscious glance. I had the sudden impression that Joe was shy.

"I think I need that one spelled out," I said, I hoped kindly. The second slice of pizza was no improvement on the first. The guard had been right. And I kept thinking about the bugs as I chewed.

He hunched his stork shoulders and sighed. "You come onto a ward—like Acute Women's—and there's all this stuff going on." He laughed. "Haven't a clue what, but there's a lot of it. And the minute we arrive, they all freeze, and whatever it was—the pattern of it?—breaks up. Just because we're there." He strode along a moment in silence. "We think we're straightening these people out. But the moment we leave the ward, it all starts up again. Whatever it was. And we haven't got a clue." He sighed again. "You know?"

I had been so busy marveling at this moody, humane discourse that I almost missed the request for reassurance. "Yeah," I said. "I think I know." In the dark of the oak tree overhead, a bird awoke and screeched loudly, once. I looked up and shivered theatrically. "Now you've got me thinking it's all a metaphor."

He ignored the gesture, caught up in his idea. "Well, it is, isn't it? Not the way the paranoids think: it's not all about us. That's the point. We're nowhere near as central as we think. But all the same, there is this huge invisible order: but we have access to it only through the grace of God."

Now it was my turn for a sidelong glance. He was gazing, his face rapt, into the lurid haze overhead. "We can't see Him." He said. "All our works just cloud the view."

We walked the rest of the way to F-Max in silence. I found myself thinking irrelevantly about Carrie B. She seemed to have something to say about Joe's view of the world, but just what exactly I couldn't catch. The connection hovered just beyond my reach.

F-Max is the one part of the complex where our master keys do not work. We waited at the door several minutes under the gaze of a video camera until a guard appeared behind the thick glass and turned a key. We followed him meekly into the guard station, where under a bank of several dozen black-and-white monitors we emptied our pockets of keys, cell phones, wallets, spare change, pens—anything that met the definition of *Contraband* spelled out on a handwritten notice taped below one of the monitors. Pizza seemed to be contraband. I left the remainder for the guards.

Past four iron gates, at the top of the stairs our escort hung back and locked us in as we walked out onto the central corridor. The doors that lined both sides had little portholes of wire-reinforced glass, and no doorknobs. At the far end of the hall, half a dozen figures were standing about. None of them was with any of the others. They watched us as we approached. Another guard ushered us into the nursing station, where the door locked behind us.

"Doc!" the nurse cried. "How have you been? Haven't seen you in weeks! You well?"

I smiled weakly. "Well enough, Lucy. You?"

"Oh, you know me, Doc." Lucy levered her two hundred pounds out of her chair and lumbered across the cramped floor to the chart rack. "Not complaining." She laughed abruptly, a harsh bray. "Not complaining." She settled into another chair beside the rack. "Unlike some people I could mention," she added. The chair creaked as she sat down, bent forward, and pulled a thick, battered binder from the rack. She pushed the chart in our direction and sniffed derisively.

"So? What's the story?"

"It's the same old bullshit."

"I thought somebody said chest pain." I opened the chart, flipped past the face sheet to the problem list.

She made a rude noise with her lips.

"Diabetes," I read, pretending to ignore her. Joe stood nodding at my elbow as I ran down the list. "Smoker." I had to squint at the next entry. "Hy Per Lip Id Emia."

Lucy laughed. "Does it mention he's a stone bastard?"

I pretended to scan the list.

"No. No, it doesn't."

"Here." Lucy swiveled to another rack. "That's 'cause you've got the wrong chart."

The chart Lucy was pulling was his psych chart. She flipped

it open, thumbed through a few pages, adjusted her glasses on the end of her nose.

"Ah. Here it is. Hmm-hmmhmm. Yeah. 'Patient states that when he locked his children in the closet, he was unable to say what exactly was concerning him.'"

She looked up over the rims of her glasses to see if we were paying attention.

"'He adds that the fire was necessary to prevent the spread of something he again is unable to identify, calling it at various times an infection, at other times a magnetic field. Even so, he states that he was aware while he was setting the fire that it would result in the death of his children. All three children died of smoke inhalation. The subject himself suffered third-degree burns to fifteen percent of his body surface area, mostly over the right side of his head and neck, apparently as he stayed within the building with his head against a wall until the wall collapsed.'"

She set the chart down. Her eyes were bright atop her chubby cheeks. "Chest pain, my ass."

"Now, Lucy," Joe said.

"Oh, Little Joe," Lucy sighed, leaning back in her chair. She directed a stagy wink at me. "Little Joe wants everyone to get better." She laughed, letting the sound trail off in a tired wheeze. "It's almost June, for crying out loud. Aren't you just about over that yet?"

Joe bit his lip and studied the chart. He turned a tabbed divider to a series of faded pink electrocardiograms. "This is from . . . two years ago. He was having an NSTEMI, I think. Yeah. Stents to the RCA and marginal oblique." He flipped a page. "But even before that he's got Q's in III and AVF." He turned the chart toward me. There were indeed Q waves in the inferior leads, evidence of an even earlier heart attack.

I turned back to Lucy. "Where is he?"

"Where do you want him?"

"How delusional is he?"

"Pshh. You want an escort?"

"Yes."

"Gary! Docs want company!" She turned back to me. "He's in the treatment room." She turned away, the chair squealing, and pushed the blue binder back in its slot.

"*Chest pain*," she said again.

The patient was a short, fat man with a moon-shaped face that was gray and sweaty.

"It's a heart attack, isn't it, Doc?" he said as we entered the treatment room. Nurse Gary, who could have filled most of the room if he had entered, remained in the doorway, which he screened entirely from the men in the hallway. A crowd was gathering.

We are not supposed to tell patients in F-Max anything. I find this hard at the best of times, but especially so when the patient is scared. "Too soon to tell," was all I could say, even though this was one of those occasions when the diagnosis is clear from the doorway.

"But it is, Doc. I can tell." His voice was high-pitched, veering toward panic.

"How can you tell?" This was Joe.

"Same pain. Same pain as last time. And the time before that."

"When was that?"

"When? When I had my heart attacks. I've had two. Don't you know that? And my cholesterol's high. And I know my diabetes is out of control. It's the food in here. It's all starch. All of it." He held out two tremulous hands, lifted his arms at either side to show us his silhouette. "Look. I just keep gaining weight. And it's all around my middle."

"Okay," I said. "Calm down."

"Calm down? I'm having a heart attack. What's wrong with you people?"

WHEN THE EMTs ARRIVED, wrestling their equipment through the doors, Lucy greeted them by name, adding, "Yeah, it's Woody again. Remember him? One who burned his house down?"

The lead tech gave her a flat stare, then turned and gave the gurney a sharp shake that dropped its wheels to the floor.

There was a tedious exchange about papers, during which the techs strapped Woody to the gurney and swung it end for end in the narrow hallway. Behind us, I became aware of several dozen figures looking on. I fought off the urge to look over my shoulder, and moved in the opposite direction, to the gurney's side.

Woody's round face shone up at me. He had oxygen on by then, but he looked even grayer.

"You okay?" I said.

He nodded nervously, but didn't say anything. He was looking up at the ceiling, lips moving soundlessly, as they wheeled him down the hall. It was pretty clear that he was praying. The thought struck me funny, briefly. Immediately thereafter I felt an inward squirm: How could I have thought that was funny? Sometimes it seems this place gets into you, and that all your reactions are becoming pathological. Sometimes it seems the real pathology is doubting yourself this way. In either case, the sensation is enough to make you hurry your steps to the next call—as if you could outrun such pursuit.

THE NEXT WAS A GUY on Acute Men's, who according to the nurse had a temperature of 106.3. There didn't seem anything else wrong, the report said, but the temperature was 106.3. This seemed unlikely, but if it was real it was probably the most acute thing on Joe's list.

The patient was seated on his bed, hands clasped between his knees, head bowed.

"Mr. Bowen?" Joe called softly from the doorway.

The face turned up. It belonged to a thin young man who couldn't have been out of his twenties. He looked at the doorway without much acknowledging us.

"It's Dr. Bellagio," Joe said in the same quiet tone. "May we come in?"

The patient made a series of spasmodic moves toward the wall that made me think of cornered prey.

"It's okay, Mr. Bowen," Joe said. "You remember me. I'm Joe Bellagio, one of the doctors."

He stared at Joe.

"How are you feeling?"

"Okay."

The matter-of-factness of his answer startled me.

"The nurse thought you might be running a fever."

The patient looked past us to the door and shook his head, miming an obscure warning.

His voice dropped to a whisper. "It's in my shoe."

"Ah," said Joe. He turned to me. "Mr. Bowen believes he has a transmitter in his shoe."

Before I could catch myself, I looked at Mr. Bowen for confirmation.

"It's not just a transmitter," he said reproachfully.

"He believes it tells him things."

Bowen's expression was almost sullen. "It does."

"Is it telling you anything now?"

Bowen cocked his head. "It's listening."

"To us?"

He shook his head.

"To you?"

Nod.

"And who do you think it is this time?"

Bowen leaned close to us, and after scanning the hallway behind us whispered: "NPR."

In spite of myself, I laughed out loud. Bowen recoiled fully into his shell, and it took Joe a long minute to coax him out.

"He's sorry. He didn't mean it. He just—" Joe looked over his shoulder at me, pleading. "He just doesn't understand."

Now I was the recipient of the reproachful stare. "I'm sorry,"

I said experimentally. Bowen dropped his gaze to the floor, where a pair of battered penny loafers lay innocently askew.

"I know," he said wearily. The eyes flickered up at me, the expression almost pleading. "But it's true. They do listen." He looked at me for a long, searching moment before turning again to the floor. "They do."

I would like to say that I said something in return that expressed my deep sympathy and understanding. That I said something that showed Mr. Bowen the error of his ways, and that through my insight he was cured. Instead I simply stared at him, feeling the empathy one feels for an insect struggling with some heavy piece of debris: cold, fascinated. A brief shiver of disgust—the same almost physical qualm I had felt on F-Max—made me turn away to Joe. I said, "Are we picking up signs of fever here?"

Joe looked startled for a moment, then recollected himself. "No. Sorry, I guess we're not."

The exam was unremarkable. Temp was 98.4.

A PATIENT ON GERO had vomited about an hour ago, which put him next on the list. At the nursing station, the unit clerk looked up from a stack of charts. "He's in the back hall."

"What happened?"

"He's been eating garbage again."

This turned out to be less figurative than I thought. The patient, an eighty-three-year-old man whose history was a scant catalog of ordinary ills ending with "frontotemporal dementia with behavioral disturbance," had been deposited here several years ago, apparently after a scuffle in his nursing home. He had a court-appointed guardian and a habit of eating out of the garbage cans.

"What does he eat out of the cans?" I asked.

The clerk looked at me. "Garbage."

I started to request specifics, but Joe explained, "We see this sometimes. It isn't food, if that's what you're asking. It's anything."

"Anything?"

"Oh, honey," the clerk said. "You don't want to know."

"Do I?" I asked Joe.

Joe shook his head. "It's pretty nasty. There's something about it—it's not just random, because he doesn't pick up stuff off the tables, you know? It has to be in the garbage can. It has to be—"

"Garbage," the clerk cut in. "Last week he yacked up a ball of tinfoil, two bottle caps, and a latex glove. And before that?" She shuddered, rolling her eyes. "Oh, honey."

"Coprophagia," Joe explained.

We found Reginald Scatliff in a back hallway. He was slumped on a low bench, leaning over a basin; a nurse sat at his side. As we approached, he retched loudly and emptily over the basin.

"He okay?" Joe asked.

"Oh, he's okay," the nurse said. She stroked what was left of Scatliff's hair back from his face. "He's just feeling a little upset," she crooned. Then, in a stage whisper: "Something he ate disagreed with him."

"Do you know what it was?"

She looked at the basin, in which a thin yellow fluid was swirling. "Not yet."

"Mr. Scatliff?" Joe called.

"Doc, you know he can't hear you."

"He can hear."

"Yeah, but he don't know what you're saying."

"Mr. Scatliff?"

The face turned upward. A few beads of sweat hung in the thin eyebrows. He seemed to look straight through us, then he rose abruptly from the bench. The nurse caught the basin as it slid from his lap. Without a backward glance Scatliff started shuffling down the hallway, stopping every ten feet or so to gaze right or left before setting off again.

We waited until he reached the next bench, halfway down the long hall, before catching up with him.

"Come on, Mr. Scatliff," Joe murmured as we steered him toward the bench. "Let's sit down."

Scatliff stood by the bench, showing no inclination to sit.

"Please sit, Mr. Scatliff."

He started off down the hall again. This time we pursued, and he picked up speed. Down at the far end of the hallway stood a trash can. We followed him as he homed in on it, his hospital-issue slippers scuffling faster as he approached his goal, his hands beginning to work at his sides. He let out a low, almost melodic moan.

He reached the garbage can and sank, painfully, to his knees.

"That's enough, Mr. Scatliff," Joe said, reaching to stop him as he groped within the can.

Scatliff glanced angrily at Joe's hand, slapped at it. He seemed to think Joe was competing with him. The moaning became a series of staccato grunts.

Joe had managed to get a hold on both wrists and was turning him, trying to be gentle but increasingly struggling as Scatliff's cries grew louder. Two aides appeared and began to lift him bodily off the floor. He milled his legs beneath him, crying out as the aides carried him to a nearby chair. When they deposited him in it he sprang up again, his eyes still on the can.

"We'll need to restrain him," Joe said. "That's fifteen minutes of paperwork. Sorry."

I watched as the aides levered him into a geri-chair. Scatliff looked hungrily past them toward the object of his desire, his head swiveling around as they turned the chair away. His mouth hung open, the tongue working over the toothless gums. In his eyes was a clear blue intensity that shone out for a moment, then was gone. He slumped back in the chair and let them wheel him toward his room.

In his room, held in bed by a Posey vest, he made no objection as we examined him. His mouth was empty, his breath foul, and from his abdomen we heard a series of booming gurgles. No response to deep palpation; no rebound, guarding, or mass. Benign.

Joe looked up at me. "Do you think we need to do something?"

I couldn't imagine anything medical that might help Mr. Scatliff. I shook myself, and made an effort to think of him as a human being who had accidentally ingested a foreign body.

"Start with a KUB," I suggested, naming a standard X-ray view that would encompass most of his digestive system.

Joe noted this down, nodding to himself as he did. He looked up from his clipboard. "Anything else?"

I looked past him at Scatliff. He was looking back in my direction, trying to see past us. His tongue swept over his sunken lips and he writhed a little against his restraints.

"Could we try feeding him?" I asked.

"You think he's hungry?"

"Worth a try, isn't it?"

Joe looked back at me. "I don't think it's that kind of hunger."

"We could try."

I realized there was something a little off in my tone: I was pleading. With what or whom, I wasn't sure. But I thought that if I could see Mr. Scatliff eating something besides garbage I would feel better.

"Never mind," I said, and stood to go. I walked out into the hallway, embarrassed. I had been thinking of Joe as someone who naively misconceived the world we live in. I didn't like revealing to him some need in me I didn't understand. It made me walk a little faster toward the exit.

IT WAS MY PAGER that went off as we were leaving Gero. I recognized the number as 1 North, Acute Women's. I traded my earlier embarrassment for pique. They shouldn't be paging me. Pages go to the intern. I showed him the numbers on the little screen. "I think this is for you."

It wasn't. They had called me because Carrie B was complaining. Shortness of breath. Tingling hands. Dizziness. Her respiratory rate was thirty-two.

"How does she look?"

This is usually a good question to ask of an experienced medical nurse, but here I could never be sure if the person I was talking to was more trained in restraint holds. I asked anyway.

The reply was clearly skeptical. "She *looks* okay. I mean, her color's good and all. I think she's just hyperventilating."

It seemed a good call. Of course, she could also be harboring a massive blood clot in her lungs. I tried to thrust that thought aside, even though I knew we were doomed to go through the full workup. Unless.

"Have you got a paper bag there?" I said into the phone. "Like a lunch sack?"

A long pause. "There's the one I brought my lunch in."

"Could you let her breathe into it? Just hold it over her mouth and nose for a minute."

Something not quite voiced that I couldn't hear. Then, "Yeah. I can do that."

"Thanks." I was pleading again. "Let her do that for a couple of minutes and see what her respiratory rate does."

Joe was looking at me, one dark eyebrow cocked.

"It might work," I said, the defensiveness tumbling out before I was aware. I caught myself. "New admit I worked up earlier. Carrie something or other. Did you hear about her?"

He rifled his sheaf of papers. "Uh-uh."

"Internal stimuli," I said. Joe just nodded.

"She's hyperventilating. Let's go down to X-ray. I ordered chest films."

Joe followed me silently toward a stairwell.

"Any idea what I'm worrying about?" I asked him, remembering that part of my role here was his instruction.

"PE?"

"Yeah," I said dolefully. Pulmonary embolism is something that happens to people after sustained inactivity, to women who are pregnant or taking birth control pills, and to people with cancer or some kind of inborn clotting disorder. It's a common cause of in-hospital deaths, and because its presentation is often subtle any suspicion usually requires a full workup. And the workup is famously mined with false results. I was not happy to be thinking about PE in the context of strange little Carrie B and her internal stimuli. There was enough I didn't understand already.

The radiology reading room was (as they often are) in the basement, where we found an empty, darkened room, with darkened view boxes lining the walls.

"Who's there?" a voice came from beyond the far end of the room. Light leaked around a corner. Reggie, the X-ray tech, appeared, and suddenly the room was flooded with light. "Hey, Doc," he said, hastily putting down a magazine. His other hand held an overloaded sandwich, which shed shreds of lettuce as he waved it in our direction. "I was just about to page you. Those films you ordered? Carrie B? You gotta see this."

An uneasiness was gathering in my chest.

Reggie whipped a set of dark transparencies from a cubby

below the counter and slapped them onto the view boxes, which flickered. Light and shadows snapped into shape.

The pair of films revealed the thoracic skeleton of an individual, young by the density of the bones, evidently female. Automatically I began to scan, following the protocol: name and date first, then bones, then—

We all involuntarily drew breath.

In half a dozen places, between the cursive sweep of the ribs I saw bright, impossibly straight fine lines, each two or three inches long. They radiated outward from the center, as if deep within the body some source of radiation spat out infinitesimal projectiles of energy. Then my perspective shifted and I realized that the objects I was seeing were pointing inward.

"Oh, my God," Joe murmured.

They were needles.

"Pretty wild, eh, Doc?" Reggie said. He waved his sandwich again. "I counted seven. There's one"—he leaned in closer—"you can't quite see. It's just about dead-on to the source. Posterior, I think. See? Right there." The sandwich indicated a distinct hyphen of light tucked under the curve of the seventh rib. "I figure she must've—" Reggie reached with his sandwich behind his back, miming a difficult stretch. "Don't see how she could've done that with all those others in there. Maybe she did that one first? What do you think?"

"My God," Joe breathed again. He was looking at the lateral projection, in which the curve of the spine stood silhouetted, the arms held up to clear the ribs.

We all stared. The image seemed to be holding itself up for us, holding its breath just as we were, all four of us in the grip of something that could not release: the shadowy substance pierced by those impossible bright spines.

"What on earth?" I heard myself slowly—carefully—let out a long breath.

"Wild," Reggie said again.

"My God," breathed Joe. "An iron maiden."

WE POUNDED DOWN the hallway to 1 North and fumbled for what seemed minutes with the keys before passing through both sets of doors. The strangeness of Joe's words was echoing in the tumult where I was unable to think: I could only feel them resonating, an unease that kept pace with me as I ran down the darkened hallway. *Iron maiden*, I kept saying to myself. *What a crazy thing to say.*

The room was dark. On the bed within we saw a shape rigid as a crusader on a tomb. It made no movement as we hung in the doorway.

"Miss B?" Joe whispered.

Only the head moved, rotating slowly to face us. The eyes were open, wide and sharply focused, giving the impression that she had been lying there staring into the dark.

The eyes returned our gaze, their surface sleeked with light from the hallway. Something in the calm directness of her expression unnerved me again, stirring up once more the inward uneasiness that had been following me around all night.

"Miss B?" Joe whispered again.

The figure on the bed did not stir. She just held us in that steady, blank stare. Slowly, as if drawn, we moved closer.

Joe reached out a hand toward her. Almost imperceptibly, she shied away.

Silence gathered, pushing back at us.

My own voice broke against it in a harsh croak.

"We've seen the X-ray," I heard it say.

The moment I said it, the tableau we had unconsciously formed began to dissolve. It was the wavering of her gaze that did it, releasing us all from the postures we had been holding. Joe and I audibly exhaled. Joe completed his gesture, his hand reaching her shoulder. "Don't move," he said.

A strange guttural sound, rhythmic and rising in pitch, emerged from deep in her throat. She was laughing. The sound rose to a high, tense giggle before cutting off with a sharp cry I could only recoil from.

I held myself carefully, suppressing the recoil out of professional habit: We do not reveal our disgust. Or fear. I kept my face as empty as possible.

"What are they?" I asked. She was taking rapid, shallow breaths, each inhalation ending in a grimace.

She took her time in answering. When she did, her voice was almost comically matter-of-fact.

"Needles."

I expected something in her expression would change, her eyes to lower, a confession of something. But nothing changed: I stood riveted in her gaze until I looked away. I focused on the movement of her ribs as she breathed. That was scary enough.

"What sort of needles?" Joe asked.

A quick giggle, quickly cut off. "I got them. Here."

"Like what the nurses use? For blood draws?"

"And injections." She nodded owlishly at Joe.

"What did you do with the hubs?" I asked.

Her gaze swept back to me, her expression annoyed.

"Why do you want to know?"

Why did I? I considered a moment.

"I'm trying to figure out how to remove them."

A smile: "I clipped them off. And pushed them. Deeper."

Joe let out a sigh and turned to me. *See?* his expression seemed to say. I wasn't certain I knew what he was inviting me to observe. Or understand. He seemed to have gotten over his astonishment. I was not any surer I understood anything.

AT A SAFE DISTANCE down the hall, Joe stopped and turned to me. He didn't need to ask the question.

"How the hell should I know?" I said irritably. "This isn't something they teach in medical school."

"Do you think she's safe?"

"You mean will she drop a lung?" I shook my head. "It's a miracle she hasn't already."

"Why do you suppose she's flinching like that?"

I stared at him.

"Do you think they're touching the pleura? Something like that?"

"How the hell should I know?" I repeated. "She just scares the daylights out of me." I turned on down the hall. "Come on. I'm sending her out."

I left it to Joe to complete the paperwork involved in the transfer. While he was working, I waited nervously for EMS.

THE THREE FIGURES OF the EMTs filled her room. I watched over their shoulders as they gently helped her stand and guided her to the gurney in the hallway. They placed her on it and began to strap her in.

"Not tight," she said. And then that uncanny giggle erupted out of her, her eyes glazing over with an inward look I could not interpret, could not even look at without disordering my thoughts.

When I looked back at her I found her gaze upon me again.

"Thank you, Doctor," she said, her expression almost prim, then catching at another inward expression of surprise as they swooped her up and away.

When I got back to the workroom, Joe was standing expectantly, pager in his hand.

"It's Gero again."

"DOC?" THE NURSE SAID. "It's Mr. Scatliff. He's vomiting and can't seem to bring it up."

I sighed. Another set of films I hadn't seen yet.

We could hear the retching all the way down the hall. There was a small crowd gathered around a bench; it parted as we approached.

Mr. Scatliff's wasted form curled over a trash can. He was clutching his gown to his chest with one hand; the other waved in the air, making a series of fluid gestures that seemed unrelated to anything else that was going on. I watched it, fascinated by its apparently independent movements. Was he gesturing to us? Conducting some internal music? The retching rose to a crescendo, and suddenly a flood of incomprehensible objects erupted from his mouth and rattled in the can.

And just as suddenly I felt, with a mixture of cold fear and uncomprehending surprise, a wave of nausea rising in me, and before I knew it I had vomited, too, right on the floor, splashing my feet and those around me.

I looked up, embarrassed. The entire crowd had turned to look at me, each expression a different mask of surprise.

But the face I found most startling was Mr. Scatliff's. He had turned from his retching to look at me, and for a moment, as his free hand wavered toward me, I imagined I caught a glimpse of something intelligent in his eyes. Whatever it was, at that moment I didn't want to know about it, and turned away as another gush of fire erupted through my chest.

AFTER AN INTERMINABLE PERIOD marked in my memory by scattered flashes—Joe's face, a mixture of concern for me and for his pager, which kept going off; the amusement on the faces of the staff; beyond them the frieze of patients caught in attitudes of surprise, incomprehension, or intense concentration on any number of objects in the area, including me; and the interminable business of cleaning up the mess I had made—I followed Joe the long distance of the hallway toward the locked doors at its end.

Radiology was dark again, Reggie by now gone home for the

night; the room flickered into light as Joe palmed the switches.
He stooped to the bins below the counter, and I heard the stiff
film jackets falling back into their bins with a hollow knock as
Joe lifted each in turn.

"Roberson, Rush, Rutledge," he muttered. "Sandler, Saknus-
sem, Scarne. Scatliff." He stood, grunting, snapped a pair of
view boxes on, and slipped the films under their clips.

A crown of ribs, translucent with age, floated above dim
clouds of bowel; a few dark pools of gas, a scatter of phlebo-
liths, the spine a gnarled tree, but no foreign body. Nothing
disrupted the ordinary shadows of an old man's belly. I let out
a sigh. Joe stepped back from the view box and ran a hand
through his hair.

"I don't see anything," I said.

He nodded.

"That's good," I said.

He gave me a sidelong glance. There was something in his
expression I couldn't read.

"How are you feeling?" he asked quietly.

"Oh, me?" I felt embarrassed again. "I'm fine."

"Good," he said, and then: "Would you mind?" He stooped
below the counter, and from the leftmost bin brought out
another film jacket. Slipping two sheets into the box beside
the one that held Scatliff's KUB, he thumbed the switch and
the images flickered into light and shadow.

It was Carrie B again. I stepped back, struggling with
annoyance. Why was he dredging this up? Below the annoyance I could feel a wave of anxiety surging back and forth.

"I think I get it," he said, as much to the films as to me.

I was beginning to feel the fatigue of the night. I could not see any connection between these two sets of films, and feared another discourse on God's mystery. I had enough craziness on my hands already.

"I think I know what she was trying to say," Joe said.

"What?" I said. It was an expression of irritation more than a question.

He gestured at Carrie B's films, its darkness hedged about by bright spines. "There's nothing there, either," he said.

I had an impulse to say something snide, but it died before I could find words for it. For a moment I wondered if I was going to vomit again.

"It's a . . . a crying out. An appeal." He was speaking more to the films than to me by now, his revelation leading him in pursuit. "She put those needles in looking for some response— not from us, from herself. Because she's empty inside, too. See?" He waved again at the films, but now he had turned his face toward me, his eyes alight in the glow of the view box, his hair a wild crest. He really did look mad.

"At least when she sticks needles into that"—he waved again without turning—"it responds. She feels *something*."

I think the expression on my face must have told him I wasn't following.

"The body," he explained. "It's important. *You* must know that."

I wasn't sure if he was addressing me as an internist, or as someone who had recently splashed the contents of his guts on the floor of the Gero unit.

"We think it's about the mind, you know. All of this"—he waved his hand in the air—"we think it's about personalities and psychology. But all that's secondary. It all . . . depends. On this." And here he turned again to the films on the wall: dark and unrevealing Mr. Scatliff, bright and mystifying Carrie B.

"It's the body that's the problem. But what makes us call *them* crazy is that they try to solve the problem: They feed it garbage. They feed it pain. The rest of us just suffer it, like the beasts of the field."

All I could think to say was, "Isn't that where we come in?" but it sounded lame as I said it.

Joe laughed. "I think we're part of the problem."

I could only stare.

"We're not solving anything. Not the way they do. Those things they do, they *mean* something. What does all our medicine *mean*?"

I realized I had no idea what he was talking about. I was tired, and didn't care. The air in the room had something in it I didn't want to acknowledge.

Joe dispelled it with a sudden laugh, a shrug. He turned back to the view box and pulled the films, jacketed them. "I do go on sometimes," he said. And then, turning, "Are you okay?"

I pretended he was speaking about my stomach, which felt empty, and told him I was.

THE TRAFFIC ON I-40 was heavy despite the lateness of the hour. I drove in the right-hand lane, too tired to join the rapid weaving of the faster lanes, pinned behind a panel van driving stolidly at sixty. I felt the trip stretching out, its duration rendered uncomfortable by my thoughts. The image of Carrie B's X-rays floated ghostly over the road ahead, the bright streaks in it seeming to crack open the darkness: something struggling to break through the shadows. I was tired of thinking about her, but the image persisted, distracting me from the road ahead. I shook myself upright, gripped the wheel tighter, tried to dispel the illusion of something hovering over the pavement, but as I did the discomfort I had been feeling, which I had thought at first was simply fatigue, and impatience over the slow pace of the van ahead, solidified, forming a solid knot in my gut.

I remembered, with a fleeting, visceral burst of shame, how I had vomited on the Gero unit. I had never done this before, I thought, not on any of the rotations of my residency or medical school, where I had witnessed things far worse than Mr. Scatliff retching up the contents of a garbage can.

What had gotten into me? The knot in my stomach would not relax: it tightened, rather, and began to burn. I began to feel as if I couldn't catch my breath. In a moment, I told myself, I would begin to feel sharp spines between my ribs.

What was the matter with me? The image of those films, the impossible sharpness intruding where there should have been only curves and soft shadows, flashed before me again. I tried to shake it away, but it persisted, and with it the pain in my belly seemed to sharpen.

I was starting to feel something more, as well, I realized: something like fear. Was I having a panic attack? Without realizing it, I had started to slow down: the rear of the panel van was receding ahead of me; lights were glaring in the rear-view mirror. I bore down on the accelerator and reluctantly, as if it, too, were laboring under some inward malaise, the car responded, the speed creeping up again to sixty, sixty-two, and the panel van drew nearer, its dull white silhouette almost blocking out the ghost of Carrie B.

But even as I tried to take command of myself, the sense of impending doom rising in my gut grew stronger, beginning to take on the unmistakable edge of fear. My pulse was accelerating. I was starting to sweat.

What was the problem? I had seen an old man vomit garbage. I had seen a woman with needles in her chest. And this had me on the verge of panic? I wasn't supposed to be scared by this kind of thing: the vicissitudes of the body hadn't *frightened* me since the first week of medical school.

It had never occurred to me before that nerve was so essential to being a doctor. What if I had lost it?

This question only added, of course, to the unidentifiable sensation still surging up in me, which I was beginning to think was the opening salvo of a psychotic break. Had I picked up something in the hospital? Some psychiatric contagion?

Unwillingly, but helpless to do anything else, I let the car drift onto the shoulder and slow down. Beside me the traffic continued to flow on, louder now as the larger vehicles passed. My hands still gripped the wheel. If I let go, I knew they would be shaking. Sweat was pouring down my face.

I tried to concentrate. What was wrong? The pain in my belly would not let me think.

And then, as the pain grew, it twisted appallingly into something that I recognized, finally, for what it was. I was about to vomit again. Right now.

I threw open the door, registering in a fleeting moment the possibility that a passing car might shear it off, and in the next moment that I didn't care as yet another burning flood burst out of me, splattering the concrete. A semi roared by, rocking the car, and I vomited again, and again, all coherent thought lost for the moment in the free fall of nausea.

The vomiting stopped, finally, leaving me bent over the sill, the seat belt still restraining me. I let it pull me back upright, putting my hands back on the wheel to steady everything, and took a deep breath.

And with that breath, to my surprise, returned not the panic and helplessness, but some access of rationality I had not expected.

The pain in my belly was gone. I felt lightened, not only of the mass of hot iron that had filled me a minute before, but of the dread that had grown out of it. Both were gone, both dispelled together, as if I had vomited up the fear as well.

For a moment I had an urge to look at the puddle on the pavement to see if there was anything there to explain this change, but the urge was ridiculous and I resisted. Because what was rapidly becoming clear to me, in what I was starting to understand would only be a brief respite, was that despite the relief of having vomited, I was still sick. I could feel the nausea returning, but with it came as well the welcome certainty that I was in the throes of a gastroenteritis, undoubtedly brought on by the stone-cold sausage pizza I had consumed so greedily two hours before. The presentation was classic.

As the nausea swelled again, the clarity of mind that had come to me with its cessation began to waver, filling with another surge that for a moment I almost mistook, again, for fear. And in that moment, finally, I understood what Scatliff's urgent gaze had been trying to convey, the meaning in those painful shafts of light scratched over Carrie B's chest films.

Joe had been right, but he had missed something as well. Scatliff's helpless gorging on what no one else could stomach, Carrie B's attempt to pin her own internal mystery: there was no special insight there, just another iteration of the problem. A problem, I finally realized, Joe shared, the F-Max nurse shared, I shared. Every patient in that hospital, and every staffer. Every patient and every doctor I had ever known.

It *is* the body that makes us crazy: our inability to interpret our corporeality, the inscrutable messages it bathes us in with every passing moment. For the patients, it wasn't their insistence on interpreting, on trying to decode those messages, that made them mad. We are no different in this. The only thing that separates them from us, I realized, is the solutions we arrive at. Sticking needles in yourself is just crazy. But do the treatments I prescribe really make a difference? Not if the problem is mind living in a body. There is no solving that.

Our bodies: inscrutable because unmeaning. They remain the essential mystery we keep trying to solve, although sanity tells us the attempt can only end in dissolution, mind and body both.

And as for spirit? Where was spirit in all of this? Or was that only another symptom, just one more fantasy conceived by consciousness out of flesh? Just then, beside the roadway, I couldn't say. Perhaps Joe could. I set the thought aside and gingerly, hoping the quivering in my guts had gone as far as it would go, I looked back over my shoulder and put the car in gear.

THE
GRAND
INQUISITOR

THIS IS A STORY I HEARD A FEW YEARS AGO, FROM A doctor who claimed he'd heard it from someone who was there when it was told originally. The story as I heard it raises doubts, however, as to when any original version might have been told. As to the truth of it, whatever there might have been originally, I doubt there was any left in the version that finally reached me. But as a story, the kind doctors might tell among themselves in the night when no one else is listening, it bears repeating at least one more time.

THE PHYSICIAN'S LOUNGE WAS not usually occupied at two a.m., but on this night an ice storm had begun as darkness set in; most of the on-call doctors in town had come in early and stayed. We staked out places on the sofas and chairs as we arrived, holding them jealously as the room filled. One of us— Benson, anesthesia—had arrived late, and now lay curled up in one corner of the floor, snorting intermittently. The room was lit by a single lamp, which left the far corners in shadow.

In the lounge chair next to the lamp sat Hawley, a pediatrician, and by far the oldest in the room. He had been long established in his practice when the rest of us began. Two of us had been his patients. A solo practitioner, he shared call with the two larger pediatric practices in town, which explained his presence that night, although some of us harbored a suspicion that he would have been here anyway: he was that kind of doctor, one of the old school that took its obligations more seriously than we do now, to the point of abandoning any life of his own. We were all a little in awe of him, a feeling tempered by the contempt younger doctors feel for the antiquated notions of the old.

We kept our distance from him, however, for another reason entirely. He was different. There was a tendency to produce outlandish statements bordering on a kind of clinical mysticism which made everyone uncomfortable, partly because he seemed oblivious to their effect on the rest of us. Or perhaps he was aware, and simply didn't give a damn. In any case, he gave every indication of thinking differently from the rest of us, and, given his seniority, and the primitive reverence his patients held him in, this difference made the rest of us nervous. No one had ever caught him in a mistake, or reading a journal.

He was also fond of telling us long, apparently pointless case histories, involving patients or practitioners who had departed this scene before most of us had been born. He offered these tales (for that was what they were, and whether based on actual cases or entirely fabricated was an open question) whether we wanted to hear them or not, and with a disregard for our obvious impatience that made the entire performance intolerable: maddening because so impervious, and so benign. It seemed mean to resent this in him, and yet we all did. Not that he noticed. In telling these stories he seemed to retreat into himself, so that his involuntary audience came to feel they had been ensnared in a novel kind of meditative practice, through which the old man sought some inner meaning that had not yet revealed itself—and clearly, as far as the exasperated auditor could tell, never would.

But what was perhaps most exasperating was that bland indifference: listening to old Hawley droning on and on, whether in the hospital coffee shop or at some random nursing station, one never got the feeling that the telling was motivated by some inner doubt or turmoil. There are cases that bother you, we all knew that, the ones that leave behind names and faces that pop out at you in the night. There's always some residue of doubt. Not with Hawley. The cases he dredged up were gruesome enough, but in telling them he seemed the embodiment of clinical equanimity. He seemed to be rehearsing the case, not in search of absolution as the rest of us would, but for some other reason entirely. It seemed—and I think this was, ultimately, why none of us could stand him—that he was telling them for our benefit.

As the night settled in more heavily around us—with the familiar call-night sensation of ill impending—you could almost hear the silent plea directed at Hawley's impassive figure. For a time, it seemed our prayers were heard. The muffled chirping of pagers became sporadic and then fell quiet, and he might have been asleep. He sat motionless in the glow of the lamp, eyes closed, facial features arrested by the light, waxen in their various droops and sags.

We had seen this before: he had an uncanny knack for sitting still like this, only to break out without warning in some interminable yarn that would not stop until it had reached its farcically implausible conclusion. He was not above claiming personal experience with spontaneous combustion. But on this unusual night as the stillness deepened it seemed possible to hope that, this once, we might be spared. We knew better, of course.

So when the old man straightened in his chair we felt both doomed and affirmed in our pessimism. He resettled his flabby white hands in his lap (hands faultlessly clean, the nails as well tended as a funeral-parlor cadaver's), and cleared his throat. Benson, the sleeping anesthetist, rolled over and moaned in a dream two words that might have been "not again."

"I knew a man," Hawley began, the formula with which most of his stories began, as immediately recognizable as "once upon a time" (and, some said, with as much relation to reality). Then, equally part of the ritual, a long pause ensued, during which Hawley could be seen to settle into himself, into whatever trance these stories of his put him into, which enabled him to go on talking in the face of any amount of indifference or contempt.

When he found his voice again, it had taken on a low, almost monotone quality. People claimed that he could speak, when he had started going at this pitch, without moving his lips, and this was what allowed him to go on at such length. Indeed on this night I had the opportunity of watching him closely, and it did seem as if the voice emerged without any movement of his face, his features lying as impassive in the lamplight as shadows on the face of the moon.

"I knew a man," he said again, seeming to have rediscovered the sentence's original direction, "who had a most unhealthy relationship with hope."

A groan made its way around the room, followed by Hawley's bland gaze. He might have been a blind man, for all the expression it held. It came to rest, blindly, benignly, on Benson. "Do you think he's sleeping?" he asked, then turned away, the question clearly of no interest, one of those mysterious flourishes that clogged up all his tales, seeming to insinuate something but in reality only inane.

"His name was—let's call him Schott. If anybody ever needed to be Schott, it would have been him. You wouldn't remember him: this all happened a long time ago. I wasn't more than a year or two out of residency. I had come back from Cambridge an apostle of light, ministering in this forsaken wilderness."

He gurgled briefly in what must have been a laugh.

"If there's anything to be said for practicing in the place where you grew up, it's that people will hold you to a certain standard of honesty. A part of that standard requires that you stay pretty much the person you've always been. In going away and coming back a doctor, I'd pushed that clause to the limit; coming back as an apostle of light just wasn't on the cards.

"But strangers were another matter, which is how this man

Schott came on the scene. He had a German name, which is nothing remarkable in these parts. But he also had a German accent, and a medical degree from the University of Göttingen, where he had also completed a residency in internal medicine, followed by a three-year research fellowship at Hopkins, in oncology.

"Why a man with that background would wind up in a backwater such as this was a question no one worried about: he was a foreigner, and that was reason enough. And besides, having an oncologist in the first place was something of a coup, the field being still in its infancy. The German accent was more of an asset than not, even though this was at a time when German still meant, for most people, Nazi. But the University of Göttingen! And the research. I think the Chamber of Commerce believed he was going to single-handedly start up some kind of institute. You actually heard people talking about the Mayo. People thought that way then.

"Schott arrived the year after I did. I didn't meet him for two or three months. Hardly anyone did. Too busy with his research was everybody's understanding, so no one resented it.

"He also had a pretty busy practice. This was back in the day when things like childhood leukemia were nothing but a death sentence. It was hard to believe that people like Schott thought they could treat it. Everyone knew you could induce remission in ALL with amethopterin, but not many people thought it was a good idea: the disease was fatal, the remissions were brief, why not let the kids die in peace? This was before Holland et al. turned the thing around. Our frame of reference had more to do with the early work on nitrogen mustards:

back then you knew, if you knew anything, that the initial discoveries came out of autopsies done on victims of gas attacks in the War. So it wasn't anything you wanted to get close to. It just had a bad aroma about it.

"In retrospect, it's amazing Schott had the nerve to get anywhere near it, what with his accent and his German degree. I think he was just tone-deaf to the whole issue. So was I, for that matter, once I discovered that I needed Schott and his German science.

"The case that brought us into contact was one of those things that happens only rarely in pediatrics, but they can make you reconsider the whole thing. A five-year-old boy, brought in by his mother for fatigue, listlessness, the whole spectrum of vague complaints that can be anything from maternal anxiety to—something bad. Which this was. The physical exam told me everything I needed to know: tachycardia, pallor, and a spleen I could feel halfway down to the pelvic brim. I patted the little fellow on the head, told his mother we would need to draw some blood, and scheduled them to come back the next day, when I was going to tell her that her child had leukemia and was going to die.

"There was no getting away from it. I was going to have to talk to that woman tomorrow, and then over the next few weeks I was going to watch that child die gasping for breath. Thinking about it, I wandered into the corridor and stood looking out the window at the parking lot.

"I didn't know for half a minute that anyone was with me until I heard a voice at my ear, soft, the accent giving it an insinuating quality that always grated on me.

"'You must have something on your mind,' it said.

"I jumped, and turned, and found myself face-to-face with Schott. He had an oddly small face, the features jammed together as though from a lifetime of looking through key-holes. His eyes had a vague, watery quality that made him look as though he ought to be wearing glasses. He nodded at the view through the window and said, 'I come here, too, myself, when it is time to think.'

"In my surprise at this sudden appearance, even more so at his peculiar insight into my inner turmoil, I leapt perhaps a little too eagerly at the coincidence of this man's appearance at that particular moment.

"'You're just the man I need to see,' I heard myself cry out, and laid before him the outline of the case.

"Schott listened to my story, nodding and pulling at his lower lip, his face mirroring my own concern. When I was done that lip curled up in a smile that made his eyes focus happily off in the distance: it gave his expression a wistfulness I hadn't expected from a German scientist, and it made me like him suddenly. 'I can help,' he said, and that made me like him even more.

"When I explained to the mother the next day just what her child had, I stumbled over my words in my hurry to get on to the good news, that there was a doctor who— And there I hung up for a moment. What was it I imagined Schott could offer her child? A cure? I had been about to say it, even though I knew that no one cured leukemia. I think I stammered up some euphemism like 'a treatment.' It was enough that when the woman hoisted up her son by one hand and followed me to Schott's consulting room, I felt I had an ally—and a ray of hope—in what would otherwise have been a dismal, lonely tragedy.

"I still remember the expression on Schott's face as I ushered the two of them into his office. We found him seated at his desk, under the impressive, black-letter German diplomas and the shelves heavy with journals and books. He stood stiffly at attention as I made the introductions, but his gaze as he shook hands so formally with the mother was all on the child at her feet, and the expression on his face was a curious thing: avid and tender and something else I couldn't identify at the moment, but which I understood later was fear.

"I didn't understand that he intended to start treating the child then and there. I didn't pick up on that part of it until the end of the day, when I got a call from Schott, letting me know he had admitted my patient for what he expected to be two weeks of chemotherapy.

"It didn't work. The child died before the two weeks were out: tumor lysis; renal failure. At the time, there were only six dialysis machines in the world, and they were all in Seattle. It's not a painful way to die. There was that, anyway.

"I was surprised at how badly Schott took it. You wouldn't have thought all that Germanic formality would have permitted the man to cry, but crying was what I found him doing in the stairwell that afternoon.

"'Ach,' he said, when I found him sobbing. 'I'm sorry.' He was actually wringing his hands. I wasn't sure who he was apologizing to, but I was afraid it was me.

"You see, I had started to have doubts, once it was clear

the treatment was going wrong, about my putting the child in
Schott's hands. I had known better. We all knew better. Leukemia was fatal. All this chemotherapy did was take a dying
child and turn its death from something tragic into something
squalid.

"But Schott's unhappiness was affecting, and at the moment
none of that crossed my mind. I laid a hand on his shoulder
and said something to the effect that he had tried, it could
have been worse, there had been some benefit. What that benefit had been I wouldn't have wanted to say: it was just the
kind of empty thing one says to a colleague in distress.

"But the effect those words had on Schott was remarkable.
He straightened, squared his shoulders, and for a moment I
thought he was going to click his heels. 'You are right,' he said.

"'With every failure, we advance our knowledge.'

"And that was all. He turned, and without another word
made his way back up the stairs.

"I didn't think of him for a while after that. But a month or
two later I heard a rumor about another one of his 'treatments.'
This one had ended spectacularly, with the patient exsangui-
nating on the threshold of the emergency room. Schott had
been there, the reports had it, wringing his hands, almost as
frantic as the child's parents, almost as much in the way. The
emergency room physician had had to physically remove him
from the scene.

"'Overinvolved' was the expression my informant used, and
we both nodded wisely. Getting emotional about a patient was
one thing. Making a public show of it was something else. But
he was a foreigner, and his specialty was inevitably a cham-

ber of horrors, so we were inclined to give him more latitude than we might have otherwise. Better him than me, we were thinking.

"The next time I ran into him was late one night, here in the hospital. I was admitting a twelve-year-old girl in DKA, and was just finishing writing up the orders when I felt something looming over my shoulder. It was Schott, standing there visibly impatient, with the hand-wringing and the sweaty face, beside himself over something.

"'I'm so glad you're here,' he started off. He looked over his shoulder. 'There is a patient,' he explained, and gestured at one of the rooms in the corner of the PICU. His expression had a guilty quality about it, as though he expected the pursuit to start up at any moment.

"The patient was another one of his treatment failures. This one was in cardiogenic shock, whether from the stress of circulating a volume that was more crystalloid than blood, or some direct toxicity of the treatment, it wasn't clear. There were some nuances to the treatment of shock in pediatric patients, he said. He would like to call a consult. But we had no pediatric cardiologist in town. Would I mind?

"Of course I didn't mind, not even when the child continued so unstable I was there in the PICU until dawn, at which point the patient went into arrest and that was it. A mercy, really, considering how things were going.

"To his credit, Schott stayed as well, even though his contributions consisted of little more than hand-wringing, and muttering in German that I assumed was prayer. And he had the goodness to call the child's parents (something I had forgotten, but then I didn't know anyone involved in this case besides Schott) and tell them to come in. They arrived in time to witness their child's last moments. Almost the last. Once the final attempt at resuscitation got under way, the nurses had to pull them out of the room.

"We left the PICU together, Schott and I. I had stayed while he broke the news to the parents, and kept him company as we both went out to the parking lot. It was early June, not yet five in the morning; the air was cool and still and dawn was just breaking. The light was crepuscular, but even so I could see Schott's features clearly when I turned to him and said, 'How many does that make?'

"You see, I had realized, as we made our way down the stairs, all this time Schott snuffling and muttering at my elbow, that I was angry. I suppose part of it was at being kept up all night on a consult I didn't think I was going to find the heart to bill anyone for. And part of it was Schott's pathetic performance. But most of it was the righteous anger anyone would feel at finding a colleague with such a trail of destruction at his heels.

"Schott stared at me for a moment, those watery eyes very wide. His expression wasn't surprise, or incomprehension. Where someone truly surprised might stiffen, he just sagged. It was clear he had been expecting something like this.

"You knew this was so because he had an answer ready to hand. 'How many?' he whispered. And those eyes of his went far away again. 'The number is seven here. With this one, eight.'

"'*Eight?*' I had been thinking it was three, at most. But

while I was choking down that number, I found myself con-
templating that little detail he had almost slipped by.

"'And elsewhere?' I demanded. 'How many before you
came here?'

"Schott stood facing me in the silent parking lot, the first
light of dawn at his back. Somewhere in the trees birds were
beginning to stir.

"'Before?' he said softly. 'Before, there was one.'

"'Only one?' I was sarcastic.

"'No,' he said, so quietly I could barely hear him over the
rising clatter of the birds. 'There was one. Who lived.'

"'*One?*' I fairly roared it.

"'One,' he said again, and as he said this pathetic little word
the sadness in his face silenced me momentarily—long enough
for him to turn and quickly walk away.

"I took all this home with me, but in the few hours I had
to get myself ready for a day in the clinic, there was no time
to think. Somewhere in the back of my mind I had a vague
notion about 'doing something.' But whenever I tried to bring
that notion out into the light of day it refused to take on any
solid form.

"What was there to do? He was an oncologist, after all:
oncology patients die. I supposed I could do some reading, see
if the regimens he'd been prescribing were at least on the level.
For all I knew he was some kind of laetrile-peddling quack,
despite the German credentials. I left for the clinic that morning with the intention of spending lunch in the hospital's tiny
library, but of course there was no time for lunch, and when

my last patient had finally left and my last note was on the chart, it was past seven. I shelved the notion for tomorrow.

"Tomorrow followed tomorrow, and I confess my intention to 'do something' languished there for months. Then a call from the father of one of my patients, a healthy if slightly accident-prone ten-year-old boy I hadn't seen since his previous birthday, dragged the whole mess back into view.

"The father's tale began in the emergency room, where Robert had been brought several months earlier with a fracture of the proximal humerus acquired while falling from a tree. In the course of the initial assessment, the admitting orthopod had ordered a routine set of films, which had revealed that Robert's fracture was only a symptom of a more serious problem. He had a Ewing's sarcoma, an extremely rare bone cancer of children.

"At that time, the treatment of choice was amputation, and the orthopod fully expected to be performing one before nightfall, until events supervened in the form of Dr. Schott.

"What he had been doing in the emergency room I do not know, and the record does not cast any light on the question either. I think Schott simply volunteered himself to Robert's parents.

"According to the father, Schott offered an alternative to amputation. As part of an investigational trial, he said, he had a drug that could be effective in Ewing's. He had been persuasive. The orthopod had been uncooperative. The parents went with Schott and his more enthusiastic view of the situation, and Robert had been scheduled for induction therapy the following day.

"And it had worked. We had no scintigraphy back then, but X-rays obtained six weeks after induction showed no tumor where the tumor had been, and once Robert had recovered from the anemia, the mucositis, and the hundred other horrors Schott's cocktail had afflicted him with, he had been up and toddling about. He had no eyebrows, and the hair that grew back in on his scalp was a 'weird, fuzzy stuff,' his father said, but they didn't care: their boy was alive, and whole.

"Two months later, Robert had begun complaining of pain in his left thigh. X-rays showed a large mass erupting out of the femur.

"At this point, the father's account grew a little sketchy. Someone had wanted to call in the orthopod, someone else had argued against it. Schott's was the only unambiguous response. He had offered another round of chemotherapy. Another experimental regimen. At which point sanity (which had been one conspicuously missing feature of the case) returned long enough for the boy's mother to suggest a call to me.

"I listened to this tale with a mixture of disbelief, embarrassment, and anger, all of it at Schott. You have to remember: this was in the days before doctors advertised. Under that dispensation, the idea of a specialist trolling for patients in the ER was hard to stomach. To advise against a necessary, possibly life-saving amputation was unconscionable. To persist in this line of approach after incontrovertible failure was unforgivable.

"I stewed about the matter overnight, and early the next morning I was in Robert's room at the hospital. I had to go see for myself.

"What I found there almost made me wish I hadn't. The

last time I'd seen Robert he'd been a robust boy just turned ten—an age I've always thought of as the very heart of childhood: old enough to have a fully developed personality, but still wholly in the light of innocence, with no shadow yet of adolescence, or anything beyond.

"That was all past for Robert. He lay there as listless as a child can be only when he's truly ill. He was cachectic, and looking even more diminished for being in an adult bed. His eyes were sunken, his mouth the angry red you see in scarlatina; I had never really seen a case of chemotherapy-induced mucositis before then. He showed no sign of recognizing me as I entered the room, only whimpered and turned away.

"It was the mother that grabbed my attention. Ordinarily, you find a parent in a kid's room at that hour of the morning, they're slumped in the bedside chair, looking almost as bad as the patient. She wasn't in the chair. She was standing at the foot of the bed, looking like she'd stood there all night. As I came in she turned and looked at me. No expression, nothing in her face, just: *See. See my son.* I felt the blood rise roaring in my ears. It was all I could do to stay in the room.

"I was about to ask, *Where is Schott?*, and was struggling to find a tone of voice somewhere on the civilized side of murderous to say it in, when the door opened at my back. I turned to find the man himself frozen in the doorway, taking in the tableau the three of us made in the room.

"His face was something of a tableau itself, registering surprise, confusion, and a sneaking guilty expression. I have no idea what my face showed; it didn't occur to me until much later that the expression on Schott's could have told me.

"We stood there, Schott and I, for much too long, before Schott cleared his throat in a complicated Germanic way, and explained to Robert's mother that his colleague and he would be consulting down the hall for a little while. Then he stepped briskly to one side, straightened his back at the door, and made a gesture as if showing me the way: a strangely military performance that made me want to wring his neck for involving me in his playacting. I felt my shoulders hunch self-consciously under the woman's gaze as I left the room.

"I held back until we had reached a vacant consult room at the end of the hall. I don't remember what I said: it was incoherent, most of it, because at that point I really didn't have much to express beyond an intense moral revulsion at what I'd just seen. Schott watched me splutter with that watery gaze of his, much calmer than I wanted him to be, and waited until I ran out of indignation.

"It was not what I thought, he told me. He had gathered enough from my expostulations to understand that I suspected him of soliciting patients in the emergency room, and I think he also sensed my skepticism about his research. As to the former, he explained that he was in fact looking to enroll subjects from the ER: that was how the protocol was written, how it had been approved; he could show it to me, if I wanted. I waved the offer aside, not sure I would recognize a protocol if I saw one. He also assured me that he was in fact named on a grant from the NCI, making this hospital a regional center for an investigation of the use of a new platinum-based compound in combination with vincristine, procarbazine, nitrogen mustard, and prednisone in the treatment of leukemia—or something like that. I may have forgotten some of the names, but that was the general idea.

"I backed away from all this chemical flummery, partly because I wasn't going to win any fights on that terrain, but also because it was all beside the point. The point, I said as acidly as I could manage, that he seemed to be missing, was that a child was being tortured. For what?

"Schott drew himself up, and his accent thickened as if to support him as he almost hissed, 'For science.'

"'You can't be serious,' I said.

"To his credit (and I have to say here that none of us gave Schott credit, not until later, when it was clear we had all underestimated this aspect of his character), Schott knew at once what I meant. He made no attempt to defend himself on the grounds of science from that moment. What he said instead surprised me. It silenced me, too, for the time.

"'Then for hope,' he said quietly. 'I give them hope.'

"I think I stood there for a full minute, unable to come up with any response to such a violent hypocrisy, before I turned and left the room.

"To this day I regret that I did not stop and see the boy and his mother, but at the time I knew I was too angry to be of any help there. Instead I stalked over to my own office in the old clinic building, and started making phone calls.

"The NCI was quite happy to confirm that Dr. Schott was indeed named as one of twenty-eight investigators on grant number such and such, for which the principal investigator was a Dr. So-and-So at the Johns Hopkins University. I called Hopkins, thinking I could kill several birds with one stone there, because that had been Schott's last port of call before he washed up here. But Hopkins was as closemouthed as Bethesda had been chatty. Dr. So-and-So was in Australia and there was no one in Baltimore authorized to comment in his absence on anything related to his research. For a while I couldn't even find anyone who would admit that Schott had completed his fellowship there. This had me going for a while, imagining that I might trip him up on something as simple as a set of false credentials. But to my disappointment I was ultimately referred to a closemouthed secretary in the heme-onc division. She could confirm that Dr. Schott had completed a fellowship there two years previously. As to anything beyond that, I might have been inquiring of a marble sepulcher.

"As I looked over the sheet of notes I had scribbled while learning so very little, it occurred to me that I might already know all I needed to get Schott bounced out of the state. He had said the project involved leukemia. Ewing's, even though it arises from an anatomically related structure, has nothing to do with the leukemias: in dragging poor Robert into his laboratory, Schott was treating something he had no license to treat, even under the lax provisions governing cancer chemotherapy then as now. In signing on to a specific research protocol, he had tied his own hands. And now, I hoped, I could use the same rope to hang him.

"I had no idea how to go about this. All I knew was that I had to get Schott out of this hospital before he killed somebody else. Because I had also learned in the course of my inquiries that in the six months since our encounter in the parking lot Schott had been involved in six more cases in which the patients, ranging in age from thirty-four months to fifteen years, had died, either from the diseases he was putatively treating, or the chemicals used in his experiments. That brought the total since his arrival to (at least) fourteen.

"The mortuary tally grew by a pathetic one the following week, when Robert, under the influence of what Schott had described to the father as 'one more cocktail,' had vomited without interruption for seventy-two hours through massive doses of prochlorperazine and phenobarbital, until a Boerhaave lesion ruptured his esophagus. It took him several hours after that to die. Two of the nurses on the case had gone on medical leave.

"When I heard this news I actually saw red. I've never experienced the sensation before or since, and at this distance it's a little astonishing to me, but it's true. As I hung up the phone my field of vision vanished in a scarlet haze. It was as if my eyes had filled with blood. Before my vision had cleared I set out in search of Schott, even though I knew it was a bad idea.

"I found him in his office on the second floor. The door hit the wall as I came through with a bang that startled me, and cracked the frosted glass. That crack was still there several years later, although by then there was a different name painted on the glass.

"He looked up, far less surprised to find me there than I was. Now what? I remember asking myself, but by then my capacity for rational reflection was severely impaired. I was seriously worried that I was going to commit an assault, which would get me into much hotter water than I had planned for him. That restrained me, enough at least to restrict my activities to waving my arms in the air.

"I accused him of a variety of things. Murder. Fraud. Violation of the Hippocratic oath got in there somewhere, and it was a measure of how serious things had gotten that neither one of us found it funny. But no matter what I flung at him, he seemed untouched by it. Not that he looked pleased with himself. He looked miserable, in fact, but not because of anything I had said. He had been that way when I arrived.

"My inability to touch him with any of my own outrage made me even wilder, so wild that eventually I couldn't say anything. I could only stand there, vibrating with suppressed violence, frustrated by my inability to change the self-pitying expression in those watery eyes.

"At last I dredged up the only thing I could think of that might get underneath whatever he was excoriating himself with: 'Have you ever helped *anybody*?' I screamed at him. I thought then, and still do, that the worst assessment a doctor could make at the end of his life would be that he had never helped anybody. I wanted to give him that at least.

"By luck, or through some instinctive understanding, I had found a lever. It left his face working visibly as whatever worm I had wakened twisted within him.

"He looked at me, recoiling as though I had offered to strike him, and lifted up a wavering hand to ward the blow. And he said again what he had said in the parking lot half a year before, only this time his tone wasn't wistful. It was beseeching. He said in a half whisper, and clearly not addressed to me, "There was one." And then his face fell apart and for a moment

I mistook the expression for imminent tears, and recoiled in disgust. But it wasn't tears.

"'Tortured' was what it was. I had never seen it before, for all the agony I had witnessed in my brief career, but I knew it when I saw it. And as that word occurred to me something else flashed through the haze still dimming my vision, cracking it into an appalling clarity. I knew what I was looking at.

"'My God,' I remember saying. 'It's the Grand Inquisitor.' All of a sudden I was thinking about Dostoyevsky. I'd never been able to make head or tail of that part of the book, but the question that introduces it had always stuck in my mind. It goes something like this: If you could usher in the Millenium—end all human suffering, forever and ever—if you could do that, but only by torturing to death a human infant, would you do it? *Could* you do it?

"I didn't understand, when I read it the first time, if there was any point to the question: it just seemed another of Dostoyevsky's grotesque Christian paradoxes. But that was before I met Schott, before I came face-to-face with someone who had also heard the question—and answered it.

"He actually rose to his feet when I said this: rose, and staggered back into the wall. I knew he understood exactly what I meant, and that he understood it because he had already had the same thought. He had made a bargain with the devil. And now had come the only thing that could make that bargain worse: he had been caught with the contract in his grasp, the ink still fresh, steaming where it stained his hands with a child's indelible blood.

"I stayed long enough to register my triumph. I had nailed

him indeed. I knew what he was, and he knew. And oddly, at that moment, that was enough for me. Far too much, as it turned out. I stayed just long enough to register the deed, and then I turned and fled that room as though the devil was after me as well.

"Two weeks later, they found Schott's body hanging from the rafters in his attic. He had been there, the coroner estimated, about two weeks: in that weather it was hard to know, but it had been that long since anyone had seen him, and the physical findings were not inconsistent with the interval."

THERE WAS A RUMBLE from the darkness behind the couch. We all turned to look as the head and shoulders of Clark, radiology, heaved themselves into view. His shock of white hair and frozen, chiseled features gave him a spectral quality.

"Cripes, Hawley," he said.

Hawley turned his gaze in that direction. His eyes were open, but the flatness of his expression made you feel he wasn't looking through them.

"Yes?" he said mildly.

"When did you say all this happened?"

A long pause. It was like waiting for some antique clockwork to perform.

"Sixty-two." He said at last. "Does it matter?"

"Yes, it matters." Clark straightened impressively. The two disheveled surgeons slumped on the couch goggled up at him. "It matters because it's all a load of crap," he said. "I came here in '64. Are you trying to tell me somebody *hanged* himself two years before that, and this is the first I've heard of it?"

He raked the rest of us with a glare that suggested we were gullible fools.

"You're filling these children's heads with lies, Hawley. None of this—" He waved a large hand in our direction. "None of this is true."

He settled back into his dark trench, muttering something we couldn't catch before falling silent.

In the stillness that followed, we all turned to look at Hawley. That bland, moonlike face beamed at us undisturbed.

"For a man who spends his days reading shadows, he's awfully definite. Don't you think?" He twinkled at us then, and I had a brief, queasy insight into why his patients were so taken with him. "What does truth have to do with it?" he said, quietly, more to himself than us. "Of course it isn't *true*. It's lies, all of it. It never really happened. I never said it did." He shook himself then, settled back in his chair, and as he sank back into his Buddha-trance we saw to our horror that he was about to start up again.

"No one knew what to make of it at first. Oh, I thought I knew—was afraid I knew. When I heard he left a note, I was afraid I might have figured in it somehow. I shouldn't have worried. The note was in German: it took the medical examiner a while to find someone who could translate it. All it said was, *I pay my debt*. And from there the whole mystery started to unravel.

"In the desk was more. A box in the lower drawer held a small collection of personal effects, the only items in the entire ill-furnished house that shed any light on the man who had maintained an existence there. There were letters, and photographs, and a few legal documents, enough to piece together a history, although as far as I know no one ever did much to substantiate it.

"There had been a wife, and a child, and it seemed both were still living back in Göttingen, although there had been no communication since Schott's coming to the States five years earlier—at which time, apparently, there had been some irrevocable rupture. There had been previous training in oncology, that much was clear from academic certificates found filed elsewhere, but there had been difficulties with licensure; it had probably been necessary to begin all over again in America.

"But the story of Schott's queer mission had its beginnings before then. There *had* been one. And as I gazed at the photograph, blurry, sunstruck, of a slight child squinting at the camera, the bald head just beginning to grow the strange fuzz of the survivor, and then at the series of later images, these much clearer, of that child grown taller, straighter, far more substantial, his head sprouting an unruly mop of otherwise ordinary hair, and of the woman hovering at his side in a half crouch of perpetual protection, I knew that I was looking at the one. His own child, who had somehow, miraculously, survived.

"Had he treated his own son? Was this how it began? And how long had it taken him, how many treatment failures followed that one impossible cure, before he had realized that he was doomed? He was doomed to go on no matter how high the numbers mounted, as doomed as the innocent victims he must torture if he was ever to pay his debt.

"How it had become a debt I thought I could understand. We are not supposed to use our gifts that way: not for ourselves. There was something illicit about it, and that first, miraculous success could only have confirmed, perversely, its essential wrongness. The only way to right the balance was to find someone for whom the cure might be an act of grace freely given, and not of selfish need. His only hope was that someday, somehow, it might all come right. Then all those victims would have died for a good reason. I could understand his thinking at least that much. Which is something else I would rather not ponder too deeply. There's enough about this case that gives me bad nights even now."

HAWLEY'S VOICE, WHICH HAD been sinking for the past hour into a half-audible whisper, finally wound down. The room was sunk in silence even thicker than the gloom. From the corner Benson's soft snores were the only sound. Everyone else, I realized, was still awake.

Hawley sat quietly for a minute, poised and introspective, before he sprang into motion with an odd abruptness, like some kind of clockwork figure whose hour had rung. He reached down and plucked an antique pager from his belt, peered at it with a puzzled expression, held it to one ear, and shook it as if it were his pocket watch and it had stopped. He stood, took a general inspection of the room, and said with a deliberate sort of inconsequentiality, "I should start my rounds. There's probably something going on."

I looked at my watch. It wasn't yet four. What rounds? I wondered. Nobody rounds at four.

Hawley took one more glance at Benson sleeping in the corner. "Somebody should wake him up," he said as he sidled toward the door. I didn't know then that this was the last time I would see him.

As soon as the door closed behind him, Benson rolled over.

"The old fraud," he said. He revealed the phone clutched in his hand. "I've been paging him for the last half hour. To his own PICU, no less. 'Start my rounds.' The old fool would rather bore us to death than see a patient."

There was a general muttering of irritable agreement, cut off when with a rush of air and activity the door was flung open. It was Jawanda from the ER, looking harried and annoyed.

"What's wrong with you idiots?" he demanded. "The paging system's been down for two hours. The whole hospital's been on PA paging but one of you geniuses turned it off in here, didn't you? Benson? It was you, wasn't it?"

Benson did what I never saw him do before or since, which was blush, and slouched quickly toward the door. Jawanda scowled over the anesthesiologist's scuttling form. "And the rest of you have three dozen patients piled up in my ER waiting to be admitted." He raked us all with vivid scorn before flinging the door shut behind him. In his wake, the lot of us sat befuddled, staring at our pagers as though they might tell us something useful, but we saw nothing that their unnaturally prolonged silence shouldn't have told us long ago.

It was close to noon before I finished my admissions. And by the time I made my way out into the world, where the ice-shattered sunlight struck me blind, I had almost forgotten everything before then.

It was only two weeks later, when the news came of Hawley's death—he had been found slumped over a chart at the Peds nursing station, a massive MI that he must have recognized, because there was an empty bottle of nitro found in one hand—that I remembered his implausible story of Schott and how he had paid his debt. At the time, I remembered it, as I imagine the rest of us did, as one last hurrah in a career memorable for little more than eccentricity. But that story, and the odd coincidence of its teller's death two weeks later, the same interval that had elapsed while Schott's body swung unnoticed in his attic, kept returning to me. It seemed to say something about how Hawley had come to be there, scribbling one of his inscrutable progress notes at two in the morning, on a night when he was not on call. There was something in Hawley's career, in its old-school devotion to service, that seemed to have about it its own element of expiation. Was there some debt he had tried to repay? I believe so, although of course by then it was too late to learn what it was, or if he had managed to settle it.

But in the years since, I've come to understand what he tried to tell us, why he chose to tell us in the way he did. It was part of that expiation, which was also why he didn't care if we thought him foolish. I understand this now, almost as well as I know how tedious you find me, now that I'm the one telling pointless stories. I don't mind. There are many mistakes we are doomed to repeat, again and again and again. This is only one of them.

ABOUT THE AUTHOR

Terrence Holt teaches and practices medicine at the University of North Carolina–Chapel Hill.